Test

"I was diagnosed with a grapefruit sized cancer tumor in my ovary and metastasis in the intestines and abdomen. The prognosis of the upcoming surgery was dark and I would most probably have to remove parts of the larger intestine and live with a colostomy bag for what was left of my life.

A few days after my diagnosis I started on the methods that Jenny has now put into this book. Since she had had cancer herself, had had success with the methods and had paved the way for a few years of research, I relaxed into the methods and got started. It felt calming and I could now focus on getting better.

The food tasted good and it felt great to actually be able to DO something instead of just hopelessly waiting.

Although I still had cancer in places, the surgery five weeks into the methods revealed that I would not need a bag at all anymore! My life expectancy had also improved considerably than what had been forecasted only weeks earlier.

I think Jenny helped me in my healing right from the start in a way that's almost beyond description. For starters the quality of my life improved by being able to relax and having a friend who knew what I was going through. (She helped me to get started with the healthy diet, which I think is important as such, but above all I gained from the mental support of a "trusted friend"). In fact I never met her before my diagnosis, but the trust was there and also her good heart that supported me in an unsentimental, but very warm manner. She was always there by my side and I can't thank her enough for her valuable support on my painful and frightening journey. Read the book. It could save your life or that of a loved one.

Sisko, Stockholm, Sweden

I felt inspired by Jenny's story. It gave me courage and understanding that there is nothing to fear. It showed me that I have another choice, that there is another Truth, and that I can take responsibility for my own health. It has been an empowering journey.

Thank you for sharing your story Jenny, and for the valuable information that gave me a roadmap when I needed it.

I. Ohana, Providence RI, USA

After a long battle with pain in joints, muscles and head, I asked my doctor for a test to be done for candida but he flat out refused. He told me I didn't have candida because he could tell just by looking at me. After obtaining the information mentioned in this book it was realized that I most probably had a severe case of candida. After following the diet and candida killing methods for a couple of months, the pain in my shoulders is gone, my headaches are almost gone, and all the other little aches and pains and symptoms that I never knew had to do with the darn candida are also gone. But most of all I can move my body and it is no longer fighting me. Needless to say, the information in this book can be very valuable also to those of us that don't have cancer but other debilitating ailments. My life has completely transformed. I am forever grateful.

Malin, Säffle, Sweden

Having worked together with Jenny for several years before she was diagnosed, I already knew that she was one of the best researchers I have ever come across. If there were anything worth knowing she would find it. Having watched her miraculous recovery I know her investigative mind gave her the right choice for healing. It has been an amazing journey to see her health blossom each step of the way. Her passion to share her knowledge and see others heal is a great gift.

Along with Jenny's insights, intuition, and experiences, she has always been able to give me invaluable ideas to help me further explore any issues with my health in order to make the right choice for myself.

Eva, Hope, Canada

I wholeheartedly recommend this book to anyone looking for hope, direction, inspiration, a guide, a friend, an answer and a new approach to living.

Tania, London, UK

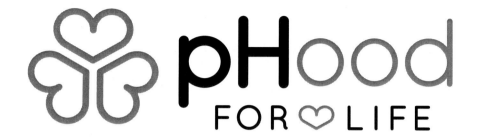

pHood
FOR ♡ LIFE

Jenny Magnusson

ISBN: 978-0-9953-3901-9 (sc)
ISBN: 978-0-9953-3900-2 (e)

Library of Congress Control Number: 2017905488

Lulu Publishing Services rev. date: 06/19/2017

Dedication

To my mother, Monica (1943–2004):

I wish I had known then what I know now.

Thank you to:

Eva: Where do I start? For being my friend, family and support

Tania: For being the ever-shining light as my coach, family and dear friend

Pappa: My rock

Donna: For always offering a safe haven in any situation

Ivana: For bringing me that first glimmer of hope with your wide knowledge in getting truly healthy

Dafna: For, through your gift, helping me navigate through the changes in me

Joe B: For helping me stand my ground

Bernice and Denise: For keeping my head above water in my darkest moment

The two church groups that prayed for me even though I wasn't even part of either of their congregations

"Let food be thy medicine."

Hippocrates, 400 BC

Contents

Note

The word **cure**

The word cure(s) has a lot of controversy attached to it when it comes to the discussion about cancer. Natural health is constantly under attack for how this word is used. One is left with the notion that the word can only be used if the illness will never return. But this, of course, can never and will never be guaranteed. When the word cure is used when talking about curing a cold for example, it is not used with the expectation that the person will never get a cold again. Below are some definitions of the word cure and it's under these definitions it has been used in this book.

Cambridge Dictionary: To make someone with an illness healthy again

English Oxford Living Dictionaries: 1. Relieve (a person or an animal) of the symptoms of a disease or condition.

Dictionary.com: noun: a means of healing or restoring to health; remedy, verb: to restore to health

Introduction

I congratulate you on your decision to take charge of your own health! The very fact that you are reading this means that you are open and curious enough to find out for yourself how one can help heal the body from cancer and other illnesses in a natural and healthy way. I am excited to share the secrets I uncovered on my journey with you. Secrets that point to that there already *is* a cure for most cancers.

But this is not just about obliterating cancer; this is about the chance to get healthier in every way, whether you have cancer or not. This is about preventing illness and changing the sick-care mentality to one of empowerment and freedom. I am not a doctor or an "expert," but my chosen work has at least taught me to ask questions until something makes sense to me...and the reasoning behind why my tumor shrank and other ailments disappeared now *does* make sense.

I hope this book can inspire you to have a discussion with yourself and spark the desire to learn more about how you can find your own right path toward better health. I have put everything I've got into spreading this important information. Many times, I wanted to give up when it felt too daunting, and it didn't make matters easier when people clearly showed their skepticism, asking questions not out of interest but in an attempt to prove me wrong by trying to expose these "crazy" methods and theories as gullible fantasies. I know I make myself a target for skepticism but I feel a duty and obligation to share the information that I have come across as it may help prevent unnecessary suffering. And to those that are skeptic about natural health: I believe it is healthy to question things but even more important to stay open minded.

But I didn't write this book to defend myself against "skeptics." And believe me, there are many. Many people don't want to believe and accept that a cure already exists (many, in fact); that this fact is being suppressed; and that, unfortunately, there is a darker side to cancer linked to certain large corporations in the name of profit. This truth is so scary and hard to grasp at first that many would rather immediately dismiss it than be open-minded enough to dig deeper and then enjoy the benefits of knowing the truth about cancer and how to fight it in a healthy way. It took me several months to accept the truth myself; earlier in my life, I would have let it go in one ear and out the other.

When I finally had this huge realization, I went through many strong emotions: shock, surprise, disbelief, anger, frustration, sadness, etc. But eventually, those emotions led to acceptance, humility, determination, awareness, elation, and, best of all, freedom, fearlessness, and health, in addition to making great discoveries about the body, mind, and soul. I could never convince a closed mind that doesn't want to know and that's not my job. I wrote this book for the very few who don't find it logical to put more toxins into an already compromised body. Who don't find it logical that a cure hasn't been found in a hundred years, when a trillion dollars have been poured into the cancer machine. Who don't find it logical that, instead, cancer rates are steadily increasing at an alarming pace. Who don't find it logical that we are still using basically the same type of treatments as we did eighty years ago, despite access to astronomical amounts of money.

I wrote it for those who are curious as to why information like this has been constantly suppressed. Those who wonder why some high-earning medical doctors choose the path of natural medicine instead, despite being stripped of their medical license, ridiculed, or even thrown in jail. Those who feel in their gut that it's more logical to *help* the body heal by providing it with what nature intended and emphasizing what the body was designed to ingest and do. There might not be many of you in an average sense, but I know that you are out there because I have met hundreds of you since I started writing this book. And I can't wait to share these secrets with you.

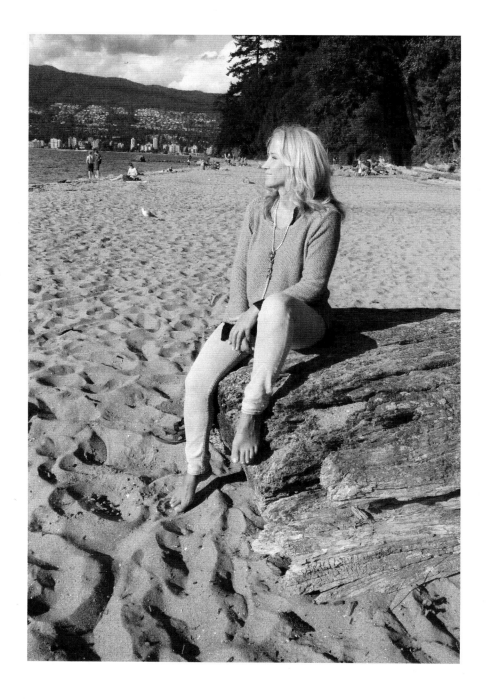

Background

I'm sure by now, most people will agree that certain toxins such as cigarette smoke and pesticides are detrimental to our health, and that the same goes for sugar and inactivity. Most also agree that exercise, stress release, and a balanced diet promote good health, increase your chances of survival, and increase your chances of not getting ill in the first place. It's a no-brainer for the public, along with most doctors. Even pharmaceutical companies and the natural side of the health world agree on this point. That all this is directly linked to health issues—even cancer—is also starting to become clear to most people. But the mechanics behind *why* that is so are rarely explained by conventional medicine, especially when it comes to cancer. And there is a reason for this.

Once you know that reason, you might start to see why conventional medicine makes cancer seem so convoluted and talks about it in such complicated medical verbiage.

I was gradually introduced to the natural methods in this book and the answers about why they work, which led to eventually discovering the shocking truth that it had been suppressed—*and why.*

Most of it didn't fall into place until *after* I had beaten my own cancer with these methods. Although I was deemed cancer-free ten weeks after my diagnosis, by no means did that mean that I was suddenly very healthy. No, that has taken years of trial and error—years of stumbling onto more supporting information and more people who have made a similar discovery in their quest for health and awareness.

I hope this book will help ease your own path to health and awareness, providing the information you'll need to get started right here, right now, while also helping you avoid errors and make better choices.

Once the understanding of the basics of cancer and how it grows is found, it's easy to accept how the body works and its amazing healing abilities.

Illogical Explanations Regarding Diet: Cancer versus Diabetes

With many other chronic illnesses, such as heart disease and diabetes, it's accepted to stress the importance of lifestyle and diet and its effects on ones' condition—but not when it comes to cancer. All of a sudden, there is massive confusion and contradiction. For example, we know that ice cream and pizza do not comprise a healthy diet, yet this is exactly what people are frequently told to eat before entering a chemotherapy treatment in order to "fatten up." We know that vitamins and minerals are necessary for a body to have optimum health, yet often one is told to stop taking *all* vitamins at diagnosis. Chemotherapy treatments, for example, help cells die (including the healthy ones), whereas nutrition helps to regenerate cells. So you are basically helping your body die a little while you are undergoing chemotherapy treatments. Does this make sense to you in the *larger* scheme of things? It won't when you find out that there are healthier ways to kill cancer without hurting the healthy cells, but instead making them even healthier.

The fact of the matter is that there is a very logical explanation as to why oxygen, hydration, detoxification, gut health, exercise, stress release, and the right nutrition would form the only cure to and prevention for many ailments and diseases, and yes, even cancer. We will explore it in this book.

Personal Experience

When embarking on my quest for recovery and health, I read numerous great books by people with impressive medical/health educations and met many conventional doctors, as well as practitioners in natural health. They had the educational knowledge and experience from patients, but what was missing for me, and what they all had in common was that (to my knowledge) none of them had actually had cancer themselves. That keen edge of knowing from personal experience was missing. This includes knowing how the body feels when going through this journey, truly understanding the challenges involved, realizing that a lot of the process is not very straightforward, and that things might feel different in an already compromised body. Given the requirements for their medical licenses, some doctors also have a limitation on what they can and cannot say. I have also met numerous people who have heard about similar alternative methods but have never actually *met* someone who tried it themselves.

So, I am just trying to add that extra layer to already existing information by sharing what I found through my own meeting with cancer, telling you about my firsthand experience, the information I came across, observations made and the theories formed.

Keep in mind, too, that most of the research that explained and supported my progress and success I found *after* I had already experienced it. Many practitioners even in the natural health field don't agree with some of this information (and often not with each other either!) but they can write their own book. ☺

Responsibility

Whenever one gets a few pages deep into alternative methods of beating cancer or chatting with people about these methods, the topic very quickly gets political. I wanted to stay away from that as much as I could, but I have realized that the facts and truths need to be expressed and that some people might not be ready or willing to enter this new way of thinking about the body and its health. This is understandable, but you, yourself, choose what you want to listen to. And with this, I am talking about both natural health *and* conventional medicine. We can't expect a doctor, whether traditional or naturopathic, to take all responsibility for someone's health, just as the doctor shouldn't be free to take the healing power of the individual away.

I, of course, strongly urge you to ask questions and do your own research. I myself was shocked when I started to put the pieces of the puzzle together and, after a few epiphanies, I was forced to go through a complete shift in thinking. This is hard to accept at first, but after one is open to it and the experience that accompanies it, there's no denying the truth. And once one has awakened to this new reality, it's impossible to go back "asleep".

Some are desperate to explain away the dramatic results that many of us have had with natural methods and natural healing theory. Others are desperate to accept the conventional explanations of why I (and others) experienced such a successful result but I now know how traumatic it is to realize that one has been kept in the dark for so long. As Mark Twain so famously said, "It's easier to fool someone than to convince them that they have been fooled." I was furious at first and blamed Big Pharma for my mother's "murder, " but then I became more accepting of the fact that this process of awakening can only be done one step at a time and by keep sharing this important information.

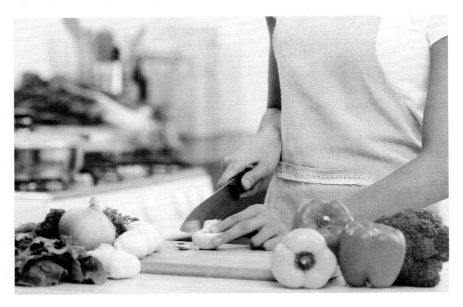

Doing It from Home!

In a study where oncologists were asked if they would go through chemotherapy if they got cancer, more than 70 percent said no. In fact, for decades, oncologists and world leaders alike have opted for natural treatment in countries such as Germany, Italy, and Mexico instead of going through the conventional treatments offered in their own countries. Fortunately, you don't necessarily have to go abroad for treatments to heal your body naturally. Most of these treatments are done from home anyway, even if you do visit a treatment center. I did mine from home with the initial aid of a holistic coach.

Remember that these methods require a lifestyle change that will have to take place at home, no matter how you're introduced to the practice. The aid of a competent natural-health practitioner is very helpful, and if you have one close by, I would strongly advise a visit for second opinions to strengthen your intuition of what resonates with you; these people typically have a much wider knowledge about nutrition than most conventional doctors will ever have.

Stumbling onto the Secret

So a few years ago I was diagnosed with cancer (breast cancer). It was the same disease my mother had died from seven years earlier after enduring a long list of painful conventional treatments. What was even more disheartening is that the tumor was in the same spot where my mother's tumor had first been detected—only mine was larger at stage 2 and was invasive, with cancer cells appearing outside of the tumor itself. At first, I thought my fate was sealed, destined to be the same as my mother's.

The prospect of walking through windowless hospital corridors for the same treatments that ended up causing secondary cancers in my mother's body and the thought of dying prematurely in a butchered body were heavy burdens I thought I just had to accept.

Little did I know that this seeming devastation was about to guide me onto a path to reclaiming my own health and experiencing a *massive* paradigm shift. I knew that I was onto something when, in just the first eight weeks of this journey, I had reduced the tumor by 80 percent without *any* conventional intervention.

As an added boon to trying to cure my cancer naturally, I also experienced the disappearance of several long-standing health challenges, including seasonal allergies, psoriasis, and a few other ailments. As you might imagine, this initial experience compelled me to keep going, building my conviction that my mother's experience with cancer need not be my own. In this book, I will explain not only how I beat my cancer with these methods, but how these other ailments were also resolved. You will find that it's part of healing the body from the inside out, instead of the outside in, and that cancer is not a localized disease but a symptom of an unbalanced environment in the whole body. Therefore, one needs to treat it "wholistically." You will notice that the explanations in this book are mostly free from medical verbiage and complicated text, as there is a very simple explanation of why these methods work.

The truth is that it's possible to stop cancer cells from growing and taking over your health—today. Yes, today! Not after a dozen expensive and painful treatments, not after several visits to numerous doctors and the bloodletting of your bank accounts. In fact, there are hundreds of natural treatments for cancer, some stronger than others. I will, of course, mostly focus on the ones I used and the theories and explanations of why they worked.

Hopefully this book will save you a lot of time spent researching and help you get started on the path to better health and a happier future. The information in this book is what I wish I had access to before my mother died of cancer in a tormented body and before I was personally faced with the dreaded words from my doctor: "So, it *is* cancer."

Once you see through the smoke screen, it's all so very clear that you can only laugh at yourself over how simple the theory really is. I am saying the *theory* is simple because implementing it is never easy. It's never easy to change one's lifestyle and even harder to be met with skepticism and sometimes ridicule, but it's sure easier than facing death. It's easier than removing body parts. It's easier than destroying vital organs. It's easier than aging too fast and losing ones hair. Let me add that for some people it's really not that challenging at all. And once it's done you are most likely left with a far healthier and happier body and mind than what you started with. In fact when one starts to address the physical body and starts to feel better, the fighting spirit gets ignited and the fear dissipates.

You might even have discoveries you could never have dreamed of. Personally, I found that as a direct result of "cleaning" the body and, therefore, also the brain, it was functioning differently and I had some profound experiences. This is a subject that deserves a lot more space than I will go into in this book, but it helps to explain of how true health works and that it isn't just limited to the body itself but extends much further. For some brilliant information on this subject check out Joe Dispenza's, or stem cell biologist, Dr. Bruce Lipton's work.

It's Never Too Late to Try

In this book, you will find steps that you can reference when starting your own journey toward a healthier—and hopefully cancer-free—life.

My hope is that the information contained here will empower you to take charge of your health and that you will find that it's never too late to at least try. You can even use many of the methods while on conventional treatments, if you choose (but be sure to check with your health care practitioner before you start).

It's true that the best chance of achieving optimal health happens with a minimally damaged body—one that has not gone through chemotherapy, surgery, or radiation—but the fact of the matter is, most people don't find out about methods like these until *after* they have been sent home by doctors saying there is nothing more they can do for them. Sadly, most people who have healed themselves naturally first encounter these methods after that heartbreaking conversation. But bear in mind that there are *many* people, even with very late-stage cancer, who have saved themselves naturally after having gone through several traditional treatments. And at the very least it can help ease some of the symptoms. So, whether you have cancer or not, whether you have gone through surgery, chemotherapy, radiation, hormones, etc. or not, please read on.

You will find that there also is a very simple, logical, and inexpensive way to kick-start the body into gear, helping it to heal itself—especially when you have cancer and, when done right, it actually starts killing cancer cells instantly!

This tool to maintaining great health, whether you have cancer or not (and the biggest secret to killing cancer) may already be sitting in your fridge and costs less than a chocolate bar.

The Basics

The "skeptic" will say: Surely we would know about a cure for cancer if it existed. The person who discovered it would win a Nobel Prize in medicine! People who recover from cancer without conventional treatments are miracles. It's inexplicable, so we call it "spontaneous remission."

It's true: Big Pharma simply refers to these "miracle cases" as "spontaneous remissions," but when something happens in thousands of people who make a drastic change and then experience dramatic results, it is no longer "spontaneous" to my mind.

Although I would call my fortunate chance encounter with natural health a miracle, the reason for my shrinking tumor was not a "miracle" and not spontaneous. And yes! Someone actually won a Nobel Price in medicine related to this particular discovery more than eighty years ago! This discovery has since been deliberately overshadowed and suppressed. More about this later.

So, beating cancer isn't a mystery to me anymore and hopefully you will feel the same after reading this book. These methods work based on the view that cancer is a *symptom* of an unbalanced environment in the body and that only focusing on the symptoms with treatments like chemotherapy, radiation, and/or hormones doesn't solve the problem in the majority of cases. If the environment and triggers stay unchanged, the symptoms (cancer) will often return.

You will find that these methods apply to most cancers. They focus on the inside-out approach and on the environment of the body, instead of behaving like conventional medicine, where the focus is localized on a specific area and, depending on that area, may be isolated as its own disease. In reality, we find that many symptoms often originate from the same problem: an unbalanced body that's overloaded with toxins. Instead of treating the symptoms, these methods focus on treating the problems that are *causing* the symptoms.

These ideas differ from the ones we have been force-fed through that sick-care mentality. Being truly healthy doesn't just mean being cancer-free or "not sick." It means having lots of energy, feeling optimistic every day, and knowing that you can achieve any goal that you set your mind to!

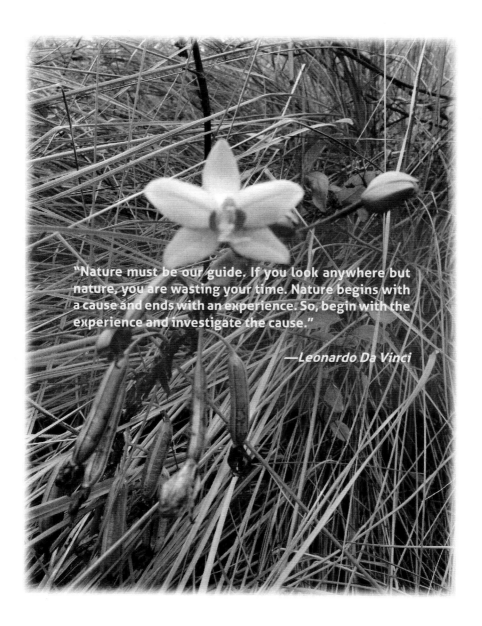

"Nature must be our guide. If you look anywhere but nature, you are wasting your time. Nature begins with a cause and ends with an experience. So, begin with the experience and investigate the cause."

—Leonardo Da Vinci

Unlocking the Secret

So how did I do it? Well, you will find that apart from doing simple things (at least, simple in comparison to chemo and radiation) like changing my diet, making sure to hydrate well, addressing my gut health, and detoxing my body, I also discovered the secret that the whole world should really be privy to:

I incorporated the natural compound of sodium bicarbonate, otherwise known as **baking soda**.

You read that right—a simple, natural product that most of us have on our kitchen shelves helped to reduce my cancerous tumor dramatically.

As you read on, you will find the explanation for why something as simple as baking soda makes so much sense when we're trying to support our health. I had repeated "aha" moments just from utilizing this first single step of the many I took to overcome my cancer and return my body to its optimal condition. It was just one of the many puzzle pieces that fell into place as I explored this subject more deeply, moving past the contrived and confusing explanations I'd always been given when I pressed for answers about my health.

The results I experienced from applying these simple, natural changes were so profound that my doctor asked me *twice* to write a book about my experience. Others, whether they had cancer or not, just had to know how I did it, what I did, and couldn't stop asking me what my secrets were.

I would encourage you to first read the book in its entirety before you start applying the steps (and, again, clear things with your doctor or health care practitioner before you make any changes). I am presenting this information from the perspective of someone who had an imbalance in their body that eventually led to cancer— because any imbalance in the body can lead to disease. So, while this book is obviously applicable to those who have or have had cancer, it can also be read as a how-to guide to help restore your body, even if you are not facing a life-changing illness. My ultimate goal is for this book to empower you to look outside the conventional medical box, and for it to inspire you to move in the direction of overall health and vibrancy.

It's important to remember that I didn't use these methods indiscriminately. It has taken years to put all the pieces of the puzzle together and create a different lifestyle for myself. It took a long time to uncover all of this information and to improve the way I dealt with my health. I guess you can say that I am entering the polishing stage now.

Five Facts about Cancer

Following are facts I frequently came across on natural health sites about cancer that I learned are key in beating this disease and other ailments that often go with it. These all have to do with changing the environment in your body. We will explore these facts in more detail but following is the short of it:

#1: No Sugar! Sugar feeds cancer. This simple fact is so often overlooked by the mainstream medical system that it is as if they are blind. A famous Nobel laureate first discovered that cancer cells have a fundamentally different metabolism than regular cells—and that they eat sugar. I'll share more about this later, but if you have a diet high in sugar, you are making it very difficult to get rid of cancer.

#2: Body pH or Acidic vs. Alkaline. Most—if not all— who have cancer also have acidic bodies. There are a number of complex processes in the body that cause the production of acids. If we get too acidic, then cellular respiration cannot happen correctly and cancer can start to grow. Cancer cells don't need to "breathe." In fact, they thrive in a low-oxygen, acidic environment—but cannot survive in an alkaline, highly oxygenated environment. (Again, a Nobel prize has been awarded related to this discovery.) Healthy cells, on the other hand, love that healthy oxygen. So balancing the body's pH levels and providing it with plenty of oxygen is essential when fighting cancer.

#3: Nutrition. It is estimated that more than 40 percent of people who die in cancer don't actually die from the cancer itself but from malnutrition. This, it is explained, is because of two primary reasons that we will talk more about in this book: 1) not supporting the body with enough nutrition and 2) nutrition being leached from the body while processing sugar. Remember that being malnourished is not the same as being underweight. Many overweight people suffer from malnutrition.

#4: Gut Health. Good digestion and healthy bacteria in the gut are vital for good health. For example, it's been discovered that many people with cancer have an overgrowth of candida, but the connection is sneered at. *Candida albicans* is a yeast that should be in balance in the gut; if it is not and the yeast becomes too prevalent, turning into fungal form, then all sorts of ailments can occur. A healthy gut is also directly linked to a healthy immune system.

#5: Immune system. Many health professionals agree that we all have cancer cells in our bodies at some point in our lives, but that these are killed by our immune system. If the immune system is compromised, it is harder for the body to deal with these rogue cells. A good immune system is vital to combating cancer, yet most cancer patients have a compromised immune system. If the immune system isn't working properly, it doesn't have the strength to detox the body and protect it against disease on its own. We need to help it along and strengthen it.

To me, it's just a no-brainer that if cancer lives in an acidic, malnourished body, one that often has a compromised gut and immune system, and feeds on sugar, you can beat it by cutting out sugar, detoxing the body, alkalizing it, providing it with nutrients and oxygen, and promoting good gut health—which is exactly what I did with these methods. Once again, it's about *changing the environment* in the body in order to make it inhospitable for the cancer.

> **"Your immune system consists of 20 trillion cells that compose your police force and garbage collectors. The immune system is responsible for killing the bad guys— any cells that are not participating in the processes of your body, including cancer, yeast, bacteria, viruses, and dead cells. 'Kill the bad guys and take out the trash.' That is what your immune system is supposed to do. But since you have cancer, something is wrong with your immune system: usually either stress, toxic burden, or malnutrition. For most people, it is a combination of all three."**
>
> *—Patrick Quillin, PhD*

Dealing with the Diagnosis

I have over the years often spoken with other cancer patients and reflected on the bad "bed manners" and even brutal way that the traditional doctors had delivered their verdicts and information and how it affected the body in the opposite way of healing. Although my family doctor later showed great interest in my surprising recovery, the way she first gave me the diagnosis was very ignorant. My friend that was with me at the time often talks about her shock in how it was delivered. I had been waiting in the drab, windowless room for over an hour and when my doctor finally showed up she just casually delivered the news before she had even closed the door behind her.

There are several tough things to deal with when you're first diagnosed. For me and, from what I've found, many like me, three of those things are:

1. The shock and realization of that: "I'm probably going to die soon...much sooner than I had anticipated...and the probability that it's going to be a painful and undignified death is also very great."
2. Sleeplessness: Waking up at 2 a.m. every night for the first few weeks and remembering "Oh, right...I've got cancer..."
3. In some ways, this next one is the most unexpected of them all: All of a sudden, a complete stranger has the ultimate power over the most intimate part of your soul - the one of fear. Sadly, many doctors abuse that power, making it very hard for us not to take the role of the victim and render us feeling powerless.

When I first was diagnosed with cancer, I couldn't bear hearing my phone ring for fear that it was more bad news from the doctors. My peace of mind was completely disrupted. I know you can't put worry out of your mind completely when you first find out you have cancer, but we need to know that in most cases, cancer does not have to be a death sentence. More often, we *do* have time and don't need to make a rushed decision.

I was diagnosed two and a half years after I first noticed a lump. It had been "missed" in two previous mammograms, although I voiced concerns about it and it was visibly sticking out of my chest. I was told it "didn't look like cancer" and that "cancer doesn't hurt." Well, mine did hurt. Even so, it was only two days after my diagnosis, in a meeting with the surgeon, that I was expected and pressured to make a decision about what to do with my body. At the very same meeting, I was told of my two immediate options: remove both breasts or do a lumpectomy and undergo radiation. I was told I had to make a decision then and there or they would have to delay my surgery date. It's crazy to expect someone to make an informed decision under such pressure, only minutes after being presented with the options! I later found out that this pressure and sense of urgency is not uncommon following a diagnosis.

I opted for a lumpectomy and then later refused to do radiation. Now, I am not telling you to refuse treatments. I am simply asking you to hear me out and then make your own decisions by following your *own* gut feeling.

When people I talk to find out that I declined radiation treatments for my cancer, they commonly ask, "Can I *do* that? Can I actually say no to a treatment that my doctor is prescribing for me?" This is a very important question. We are often rushed into making uninformed decisions about matters as important as removing body parts or even vital organs. These are not decisions to be made haphazardly—far from it— do your research and follow your heart and gut. If you feel pushed, ask for a moment to think about it. Your friends and loved ones might also put pressure on you to follow the doctors' advice. This is understandable, as they only want what they think is best for you and are probably panicking as much as you are (if not more). But it is *your* choice. Whatever you choose to do, you will have a better chance to battle the cancer if you believe in your treatment. Needless to say, I didn't believe in the treatments prescribed for me, as my mother died despite doing everything the doctors told her. This experience put me in a better position to be skeptical about conventional treatments. It took me a long time to understand the holistic side of healing and how it would relate to my particular situation. In hindsight I can see why I couldn't expect others to give me informed advice of what I should do and why I shouldn't blindly follow it.

A (Simple) Comparison

First a look at my mother's case:

My mom was diagnosed with breast cancer. Eight years later, she died with cancer found all through her body. During these eight years, she had several surgeries and went through aggressive radiation, chemotherapy, and hormone treatments. Toward the end, her lungs ran at 20 percent of their capacity. Her heart was damaged and her thyroid was wiped out. She had joint problems and stomach problems, and she couldn't swallow properly. The list goes on and on...

The only nutritional advice given to my mother was not to worry about food and that it's ok to go ahead and eat chocolate and drink wine. This nutritional "advice" is still frequently given today to patients around the world.

After taking a hard look at the picture of my mom, I came to realize that it didn't help to merely address the cancer in her breast, as it showed up throughout her whole body in the end and she died. I also came to realize that most of her body's collapse didn't come from the cancer itself but from the effects of the "treatments" she had gone through.

Now to my body:

I was diagnosed with stage II invasive ductal carcinoma with cancer cells outside of the tumor. The tumor was found in almost exactly the same spot as my mother's first cancer was discovered, only mine was larger. I also had pretty bad seasonal allergies, eczema, a runny/stuffy nose, severe fatigue, mood swings, sugar cravings, and other ailments that I later understood were all connected to my "condition"—an acidic, unbalanced body. Some of those symptoms were also true in my mother's case.

Now, I was lucky enough to know of a holistic coach/blood analyst who I went to just a few days after my diagnosis. In a daze, and still in shock I thought that my mom's fate would also be mine. The holistic coach gave me some great, reassuring advice, expounded on some theories, and gave me tools to get started. This first contact with natural health was a game changer. It was soothing and non-threatening. I felt safe enough to start to investigate further.

This is where the road to recovery, health, and, freedom began. From this basis, I uncovered the 12 steps I used to rid myself of cancer and restore my health. Remember, you may not have the same results, as we are all different people with different health histories, different health issues, and different levels of severity of these issues. It simply means that this path worked for me and many others, and that it could work for you, too. We will revisit this comparison with the results later in the book.

> **"If the fish is sick, what would you do? Treat the fish or change the water?"**
>
> *— Robert O. Young, PhD (author "The pH Miracle")*

And if one takes a sick fish out of a dirty fish tank and treats it, one doesn't put that fish right back in the dirty tank again. So why do this to a cancer patient?

Viewed that way, the secret to getting healthy is simple—change the **environment**.

I've used the following steps to do just that, changing the environment within my own body to promote health and wellness.

12 Steps to Health

1

pH Balance

This first step is, in my view, the most important one. It will help you understand how recovery from cancer through these natural treatments works and to get an overall understanding of how the body responds.

Learning to balance your pH *teaches* and *forces* you onto the right path in the areas you need to address next. This is where the path to health started for me.

We will talk more about why something like this very vital knowledge about pH has been kept quiet later on in the book. For now, let's focus on the discovery itself and what it provides in supporting these methods. This might be the most important information of all in unlocking good health, and it won't be kept secret from you anymore.

In 1931, Otto Warburg won the Nobel Prize in medicine for his discovery that cancer cells cannot survive in an alkaline and highly oxygenated environment. The methods in this book are based on this crucial discovery.

At a lecture in 1966, Warburg said, "Cancer, above all other diseases, has countless secondary causes. But even for cancer, there is only one prime cause, summarized in a few words: the prime cause of cancer is the replacement of the respiration of oxygen in normal cells by a fermentation of sugar."

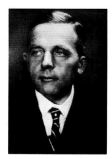

Otto Warburg

1

In other words: cancer lives by *not* breathing in an acidic environment, but rather feeding on sugar (which includes the glucose that the body releases while stressed). Healthy cells grow by provision of oxygen, whereas cancer cells grow through provision of sugar but *die* by the provision of oxygen and alkalinity.

So, based on these discoveries we have now established that cancer thrives in an acidic environment (low pH) but dies in an alkaline environment (high pH).

It is very simple: if cancer cells cannot survive in an alkaline and highly oxygenated environment, we can kill those cancer cells by providing that ideal environment in the body.

The pH (potential hydrogen) scale measures how acidic or alkaline (basic) a substance is, including our own bodies. It ranges from 0 to 14. 7 is neutral; above 7 is alkaline and below 7 is acidic. The human body should be slightly alkaline, with a pH in the range of 7.2–7.4 for optimum health. Studies have shown that most, if not all, cancer patients have an acidic body. One important note: for those of you reading who have not been diagnosed with cancer, just because you have an acidic body it doesn't by any means mean that you might have cancer. What it does mean, though, is that your acidic body provides an environment in which certain diseases and ailments thrive; that potentially includes cancer. It is also difficult for an acidic body to absorb nutrients. So maintaining a healthy pH and a healthy environment in the body helps to prevent illness.

(Quote from Dave Mihalovic "Prevent Disease.com" in article on "Baking soda cancer treatment": "When the body can no longer effectively neutralize and eliminate the acids, it relocates them within the body's extra-cellular fluids and connective tissue cells, directly compromising cellular integrity.")

According to Dr. Mark Sircus, "All cancer sufferers, and, in fact, every chronic disease patient should hold clearly in mind that pH is a regulatory authority that controls most cellular processes. The pH balance of the human bloodstream is recognized by medical physiology texts as one of the most important biochemical balances (Sircus 10)."

Obviously, pH is important. But how do you know if your body is too acidic?

Testing Your pH

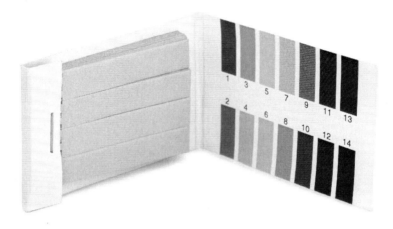

There are different ways to test your pH, helping guide you to achieving healthy levels. One way, and perhaps the most accurate, is to have your blood tested at a lab. In my case, it was established that my blood was extremely acidic. It's not necessary to have a blood test done to test your pH, though. The easiest and most common method is to test your saliva or urine using a piece of litmus paper. This little piece of paper will change colour based on the pH of the liquid it touches, most commonly turning yellow, green, grey, and blue. Blue is normally the desired range, as it indicates an alkaline environment in the body, but some tests use a different colour scheme. I had a blood test done at the blood analyst's office, but then used litmus paper after that to continue testing as I embarked on my 12 Steps to health. pH testing litmus paper normally costs around $15 in health food stores, but you might find packets cheaper online.

At first, I was so acidic that the colour of the litmus paper didn't even change.

The "Monitoring Device"

Testing your pH levels regularly is vital to employing the methods in this book. Apart from telling you whether you need to balance your levels, it also helps you learn to get in tune with your body overall. I think of this as the "monitoring device" for health. I went through a period of very low readings (acidic), although I felt I was doing everything right: drinking plenty of water, eating a very alkaline diet, etc. My low readings told me that something else needed to be addressed and it was suggested that I try to increase my intake of healthy fats. I increased my Omega-3 oil intake and sure enough, my readings quickly went up. Why? Because the body needs healthy fats in order to properly absorb the nutrients that you provide it. More about healthy oils and fats in the step addressing nutrition (#5).

So can scenarios like this explain why similar diets and methods work on some people, but not on others? I believe that for some, diet alone may not raise the pH to a healthy level. And if the pH levels were not regularly measured, they would be unaware that they were not making enough progress toward becoming more alkaline. Many things can affect your pH levels: having been stressed about something the day before, not hydrated enough, having drunk alcohol or coffee before testing, testing your urine first thing in the morning when the body is naturally more acidic, and so on. Because of this, you should test yourself a few times to help get a sense of how acidic you actually are. Always test well after meals, as this also will affect your readings.

I am intrigued by stories of the native Inuit people, who were virtually cancer-free until a "Western" lifestyle reached them. Although they didn't eat many alkalinizing vegetables and fruit, they still got plenty of fresh air and exercise. They ate no sugar or dairy, drank no alcohol, and lived reasonably low-stress lives in a tight-knit community. They also enjoyed healthy fats from eating salmon, whale meat, and seal blubber. These conditions would have all added up to having an alkaline body and therefore a lower risk of cancer.

Sodium Bicarbonate (Baking Soda, NaHCO$_3$)

> "Cancerous tissues are acidic, whereas healthy tissues are alkaline. At a pH slightly above 7.4, cancer cells become dormant and at pH 8.5, cancer cells will die while healthy cells will live. This has given rise to a variety of treatments based on increasing the alkalinity of the tissues such as a vegetarian diet, the drinking of fresh fruit and vegetable juices, and dietary supplementation with alkaline minerals such as calcium, potassium, magnesium, cesium, and rubidium. But nothing can compare to the instant alkalinizing power of sodium bicarbonate for safe and effective treatment of cancer."
>
> — *Mark Sircus Ac., OMD, director of the International Medical Veritas Association*

Now that you know about the body's need for a balanced, slightly alkaline pH, it's time to talk about one of the most important secrets regarding cancer recovery and treatment. This is where it essentially all started for me: sodium bicarbonate or baking soda (and just to be clear, we are talking baking *soda* and not baking *powder*).

Yes, that same baking soda that can clean out your kitchen sinks, get rid of unpleasant smells caused by pets or rotting food, or make your skin exceptionally soft when you add it to your bath water helps to increase your alkalinity.

The benefits of sodium bicarbonate are so extensive that there are several books on the subject. Here, I will give you a brief introduction; you can research further on your own (I highly recommend Dr. Mark Sircus's books on sodium bicarbonate).

If I had cancer and had no access to any nutritious veggies or fruit, supplements, or oils, and was bedridden, there are two things I would do: hydrate with plenty of pure water and take baking soda for a couple of weeks. Here's why:

Sodium bicarbonate is one of the fastest working natural substances that can help right the wrongs we do to ourselves and kick-start our bodies to better health. It is completely harmless as long as it is taken properly (and isn't that always the case?). If not taken properly, there have been reports on issues—for example, if taken in huge amounts, it has been said that it may cause an interruption in nerve signals to the heart (although I have also read this is not true), that it could damage certain tissues in the body and I heard that there has also been a report of stomach rupture and that this could happen if taken too soon after a meal and in excessively large quantities. I have never met or talked to anyone or read any specific evidence on the matter, but it is something to still consider when starting *any* treatment; there may be some sort of risk factor. But think about the known risks of conventional treatments, where the vast majority of patients will experience some type of side effect and a lot of people have their cancer return or die of complications and consequences connected to those treatments. Personally, it was a no-brainer to try the baking soda. So let's keep things in perspective: if taken properly, there are few to no side effects to taking sodium bicarbonate. Instead, it is actually healthy for the body.

Sodium bicarbonate is a type of salt that's found naturally in the earth and in our bodies. In fact, the job of sodium bicarbonate in our bodies is to balance pH levels! But because of the gradual depletion of sodium bicarbonate in modern agriculture, most of us don't get enough of it through our diet anymore. It is therefor frequently suggested for anyone to occasionally take a little bit of sodium bicarbonate to boost the system even when not dealing with severe health problems.

This natural salt has a dramatically high pH. It cannot be patented because it occurs without any biotechnological or pharmaceutical intervention—hence the controversy surrounding this natural and inexpensive salt and why it is being kept secret.

When you consider its benefits and realize that baking soda is incredibly cheap, it is no wonder that the pharmaceutical companies frown on its use—for mere pennies, people can start to change their body's alkalinity and begin shrinking cancerous tumors. One package of baking soda is usually enough to last through your treatment if taken orally.

You can't get chemotherapy, even in "small doses," without killing healthy cells that help your body function. In contrast, baking soda helps the body start healing without killing anything useful; in fact, it makes the body inhospitable to candida and other pathogens that might make us sick. There are many brands of baking soda you can take and I don't specifically recommend any particular one. I can tell you what worked for me, though.

I was first recommended to take Pleo-Alkala powder, which is a product manufactured in Germany and sold as an antacid. Alkala is sodium bicarbonate—baking soda—with some added potassium, which is also beneficial for the body. This worked well for me, but I started using plain baking soda after I learned that it was essentially the same and had similar effects. I suggest using a brand that doesn't contain aluminum; other than that, one isn't necessarily better than any other. Most health food stores should carry aluminum-free baking soda. I mostly used Arm & Hammer, though I used a different brand for a while after hearing rumors that it contained aluminum; I have since found out that this is not the case.

My baking soda routine

I started by testing my urine before breakfast and would take a scoop of Alkala (or a teaspoon of baking soda) in a glass of water an hour after breakfast. It's important to note here that I tested myself on the second urination in the morning, since the first one is usually acidic from toxins that have accumulated in the body overnight. If you test alkaline first thing in the morning, it could mean that these toxins are not being eliminated properly, but if this happens while on the baking soda regimen (which it did in my case), it might be because the baking soda is so very alkalizing. My readings changed back to normal (slightly acidic first thing in the morning) when I stopped taking the baking soda treatment.

If I was still acidic when I tested myself before lunch, I would take another teaspoon of baking soda in a glass of water between lunch and dinner. It's important to take the baking soda away from meals, as you need your stomach acids to digest the food (a side effect of taking baking soda too close to a meal could be bloating and gas).

The intake of baking soda kick-starts the body to take up more oxygen and alkalize the blood.

Following this routine is recommended for only two to three weeks. By then, you should be up and running, raising your body's pH naturally through diet, oxygen, hydration, etc. In other words, you should be supporting the ways your body would normally alkalize itself if it wasn't overly toxic from a poor diet, environmental toxins, stress, and so on.

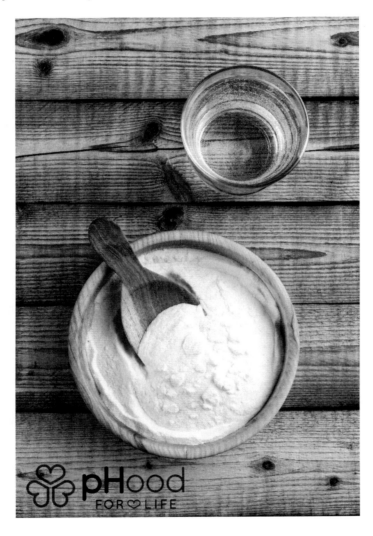

I alkalized my body aggressively with baking soda the first couple of weeks, but then eased down once I learned how to alkalize my body without the aid of sodium bicarbonate. I still occasionally use a teaspoon of baking soda here and there when I feel I need a boost, but it's very rare these days, as I have become quite good at adjusting my body pH in other ways. In any case, you should try not to aggressively use sodium bicarbonate for more than three weeks. Should you still have challenges raising your pH after three weeks or if you have problems ingesting the sodium bicarbonate, try using a quarter-cup of it in your bath water. The skin absorbs the sodium bicarbonate and, as a bonus, makes your skin silky-soft. Should you also have skin problems such as psoriasis or eczema, it helps soothe the skin.

It's important to mention that, yes, there could be a danger in being too alkaline for too long. This is why you only use baking soda to correct the initial imbalance, and then start to make the lifestyle changes that are mentioned in this book, like reducing stress, eating better, and so on, allowing your body to alkalize itself on its own. Sodium bicarbonate raises the pH aggressively. If you are too alkaline for too long, you might notice some side effects (and there has been suggestions of increased mold, fungus and yeast if too alkaline for too long), but when taken for a shorter period of time and in moderation, baking soda can be a great help.

How much is too much? I myself took one teaspoon twice daily for two to three weeks, but have come across other people who have taken larger dozes and for a longer period without any negative effects. Pay attention to your body and start implementing lifestyle changes right away; that's the best way to move toward optimum health.

In short, baking soda provides emergency care for the initial symptoms (e.g., a tumor), but the actual problem that has caused these symptoms still needs to be addressed.

Another reason you only want to use the baking soda as a "kick-start" method and not for an extended period is because the body will sometimes try to balance an overly alkaline environment by attempting to acidify it again. Because of this mechanism, you could yo-yo a lot in the beginning. It is not easy, but don't lose faith if you struggle a bit. It takes a bit of time to get to know how your body responds, but with time, attention, and monitoring, you'll figure it out—and in the process, it's likely you will quickly see some dramatic benefits to your overall health.

A misconception about salt

Sodium bicarbonate is a type of salt, so you might be thinking, "but I thought salt was bad for you." After studying this subject further, I realized that this is not true; the body *needs* a certain amount of salts to function properly. When it gets problematic is when we *overuse* salts and, most importantly, use the *wrong kind* of salt. Himalayan pink salt, for example, is an excellent source of salt that also contains healthy minerals such as magnesium, potassium, and calcium, as does good sea salt. Because of its minimal processing, sea salt retains many of its minerals and has no added ingredients. Table salt, on the other hand is often stripped of its minerals and many contain added chemicals such as anti-caking agents.

Sea salt also contains iodine, which our bodies need for thyroid health. Iodine has great results in combating psoriasis and protects the thyroid against radiation—hence the strong demand for iodine in stores following the Fukishima disaster.

The misconception that all salt is bad for us may also explain why certain natural methods that exclude sodium, though they may have some success through detoxification and improved general nutrition, don't always have an optimum effect on recovery—they don't include healthy levels of salt. Salt in the right amounts have helped me stay hydrated as it makes the body retain more fluid. Taking in moderate amounts of salts that include healthy minerals, such as Himalayan salt or minimally processed sea salt, as well as sodium bicarbonate, have been an important part of my recovery.

Dr. Sircus: "Sodium bicarbonate acts as a powerful, natural, and safe antifungal agent which, when combined with iodine, covers the entire spectrum of microbial organisms." It has also been attributed as being effective in combating candida (more on this later). It's worth mentioning, too, that some athletes even use sodium bicarbonate to reduce the lactic acid in their bodies, and some women use baking soda to treat their yeast infections. Since it reduces the acids in the body, it naturally aids in reducing acid reflux. And its uses don't end there. There are more than a hundred uses for sodium bicarbonate.

Placebo effect

Sodium bicarbonate is so powerful that pharmaceutical companies, cancer agencies, and nonprofit organizations supposedly looking for a cancer cure try their best to hide its efficacy by creating an air of ridicule around it and those who advocate its use. They try to explain away the successes seen with it by saying it is simply a placebo. Now, let's think about this for a moment. The definition of the placebo effect reads: "A beneficial effect, produced by a placebo drug or treatment, that cannot be attributed to the properties of the placebo itself, and must therefore be due to the patient's belief in that treatment."

In other words, if you really believe that something will work, it does. So, if that is the only case they are arguing, shouldn't the same work for their chemo drugs? In fact, shouldn't it work way *better* with chemo drugs, since we are enthusiastically "allowed" to believe in them, and the belief in them is strongly supported by these charities that most people tend to put their trust in? If you believe in chemo drugs, you will not be ridiculed. You will have the full emotional support of your friends and family, and especially of the medical establishment. The fact that Big Pharma is suggesting that baking soda works due to the placebo effect is incredibly good news, because this means that they are actually accepting the placebo effect as real. Let's be logical. If the placebo effect is real and that is the only thing at play when people have dramatic results from taking baking soda and "melting" their tumors away, does it really matter? Does it change the results if you call it a placebo effect instead of a treatment or cure? No, of course not. Even if these results are explained as simply as being part of the placebo effect, those results would be reason enough to try this technique.

But dig deeper. I'm not on board with the concept that sodium bicarbonate is merely a placebo. For it to be a placebo, you would have to really believe that this substance would truly help. That wasn't the case when I tried it. During the first five weeks I tried these methods, I was in a mental vacuum; I didn't know what to believe. I was in shock and very confused. I *did* take baking soda, but I didn't yet know why it would be so beneficial—or whether it would be beneficial at all. After the first five weeks, my tumor had shrunk to almost half its original size (and then another 30% from its original size over the following three weeks). I'd hardly call that a placebo...or luck...or a miracle...or a "spontaneous remission" (the most ridiculous conventional excuse for the success of natural treatments against cancer). Furthermore, when the establishment tries to explain away the power of baking soda, it's often claimed that no study has proven its effectiveness or its mechanism. This is not true.

Nowadays I just shake my head at these desperate ways of trying to explain away baking soda's effectiveness. The real reason is very simple: it raises the pH. It helps the cells take up oxygen. Cancer dies in a highly alkaline and oxygenated environment. End of story.

Dave Mihalovic: "A 2009 study published in the journal *Cancer Research* is among the first to confirm that the alkalizing effect of sodium bicarbonate can indeed stop cancer. By injecting bicarbonate into a group of mice, the authors of the study were able to determine how the growth and spread of cancer tumors were affected by raising the pH of the organ affected by the cancer. The study results showed that baking soda indeed raised the pH and reduced spontaneous metastases in mice induced with breast cancer. The researchers also determined that sodium bicarbonate works by raising the pH outside the cells and not within cells. This is an important finding because it suggests that sodium bicarbonate does not interfere with cellular metabolism even as it makes the microenvironment unconducive for tumor growth."

> **"Cancer seems to grow slowly in a highly acid environment (because the acids cause it to partially destroy itself) and may actually grow more quickly as your body becomes more alkaline prior to reaching the healthy pH slightly above 7.4 where the cancer becomes dormant. Therefore, it is important to get pH above 7.4 quickly."**
>
> *— Mark Sircus Ac., OMD, director of the International Medical Veritas Association*

Dr. Sircus's account is the only one I have come across regarding the importance of quickly reaching an alkaline state. I find his findings very interesting, though, and worth mentioning, since his theories would explain why cancer grows more quickly in some people as opposed to others. I had a very acidic body when diagnosed and my cancer was slow-growing. I got my body up to aggressively alkaline levels most of the time during my first two weeks using sodium bicarbonate, but was also very acidic some days; I yo-yoed a bit before eventually learning to keep my alkalinity levels right using only food. Although the information on the importance of becoming alkaline quickly is interesting and sounds plausible, I think it's important to not panic when learning to get your pH levels up. If combined with other steps, any movement toward a more alkaline environment will help your body to heal. For instance, the nutrition you provide your body with helps to stop the body from leaching nutrients from tissue and organs. And remember that the body needs a certain amount of acid to digest that healthy food you're eating.

As mentioned, sodium bicarbonate has many uses and benefits. One of the less-known facts about baking soda is that it is used in emergency medicine and has even been used in cancer patients for years by conventional oncologists; they sometimes inject patients with sodium bicarbonate to protect the kidneys before administering chemo drugs.

Should you want to find out more about the many wonderful uses of sodium bicarbonate and the many secrets surrounding it, be sure to read Dr. Mark Sircus's fascinating book, *Sodium Bicarbonate, Nature's Unique First Aid Remedy.* This book gave me quite a few insights into this useful substance. For instance: "It has blood vessel dilating action (vasodilator), increases blood fluidity, facilitates blood flow delivery as well as assisting oxygen dissociation from hemoglobin—thus, more oxygen flows to the capillaries and cells. Through the 'Bohr Effect,' more oxygen is released from hemoglobin. Bicarbonate also has strong anti-inflammatory action,,helps with detoxification and neutralization of toxic substances of all kinds, offering strong and almost instantaneous shifts in pH."

Sircus's work with sodium bicarbonate began when he found out that bicarbonate was used by the Army in cases of uranium exposure to protect the kidneys and after hearing about Dr. Tullio Simoncini's work (we'll get more into that later). Dr. Sircus has been particularly interested in its use with cancer patients and has written the book *Rich Man's Poor Man's Cancer Treatment.*

Again, let me stress that I read Dr. Sircus's book years after my successes with sodium bicarbonate; this information didn't help make baking soda some kind of placebo for me. It only made my conviction stronger of its beneficial action and that it's more than worth trying for yourself.

As always, be sure to tell your health provider if you want to use sodium bicarbonate as part of your healing process.

Summary:

The human body should have a pH in the range of 7.2–7.4 for optimal health.

It is believed that most, if not all, cancer patients have acidic bodies.

Test your pH levels regularly. Always test away from meals. Keep in mind to test your second urination if testing your urine in the morning.

Litmus paper can be acquired online or at certain health food stores and naturopathic offices.

Taking sodium bicarbonate correctly helps kick-start the oxygen uptake and increases pH levels.

Should you want to use sodium bicarbonate like I did, take one teaspoon in a glass of water twice a day, away from meals. Try not to use it like this for more than two to three weeks.

2

No to Sugar! Sugar Feeds Cancer

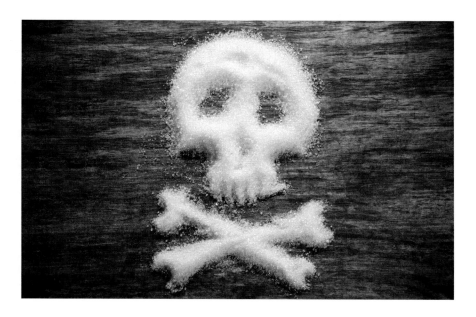

The next step in learning how to balance your body is to eliminate sugar as best you can. Sugar feeds cancer.

There's no denying it. Sugar is even used to detect cancer. No biologist with a good conscience will tell you otherwise.

Cutting out sugar is critical when fighting cancer. No more refined sugar, pop, alcohol, or desserts; even certain fruits and fruit juices are too sweet in the initial stages of combating cancer. Most of these sugary foods and drinks are also the most acid-forming foods on the scale.

I eventually learned where the "hidden" sugars were and tried to avoid those as well. The best guide to follow is to try to **stay away from**

anything that ends with –ose. That includes sucrose (pasta, bread, etc.); fructose (certain fruits are too sweet at first, although pears, apples, and berries are fine); lactose (dairy such as milk; milk is also mucus-forming); glucose (more glucose is released from the liver when stressed, which is why stress reduction is so important); and maltose (bread).

When I wanted something sweet, I used Stevia, a natural alkalizing herb that regulates blood sugar.

Raw honey, pure maple syrup, and molasses are also healthy and nutritious sweeteners when used in moderation and I started using them occasionally as my body found balance again. Raw honey contains healthy enzymes, while molasses contains more calcium than milk and is a rich source of potassium, so they are actually quite good for you in moderation. There are other natural sweeteners that have popped up on the market such as monk fruit and coconut sugar/syrup that one can try when ready for sweeter additions to the diet.

You'll want to avoid artificial sweeteners such as aspartame as these have been proven harmful to ones health. If you do use dairy products such as yoghurt, opt for full- fat, organic, natural products and choose the ones without added flavor. Stay away from those with labels such as "fat- free," as they often contain harmful ingredients— including sugar. A good alternative to yoghurt from dairy is goat's milk yoghurt or sheep's milk yoghurt.

But there are a few dairy products that actually are beneficial for the body even when fighting cancer, such as butter and cottage cheese. Butter is alkalizing and cottage cheese helps fight cancer if blended with flax oil. This use is called the "Budwig protocol."

Another frequently overlooked source of sugar is alcohol. Though some beers and wines do contain beneficial ingredients, such as hops or resveratrol, they are mostly just fermented sugar. The minute alcohol reaches the bloodstream, the body, responds to it as if you just drank a big glass of sugar-filled soda or fruit juice. Some claim it's a myth that alcohol turns to sugar when you digest it, but even so, your body undergoes undue stress when drinking, as the liver works to break that alcohol down into carbon dioxide and water. In the body, alcohol is essentially treated as a toxin. The liver becomes preoccupied with breaking down the alcohol and cannot properly metabolize the nutrients your body needs—especially if you are fighting cancer. Alcohol is also extremely acidic. It is best to steer clear of alcohol altogether while you're balancing the body back to a healthy state again. As a side benefit, many people lose unwanted pounds when they cut down or eliminate alcohol because it contains a very high amount of empty calories and little real nutrition.

I know these changes may sound daunting, but it does get easier as you get past the first couple of weeks of sugar cravings. Your body responds to sugar in much the same way a cocaine addict's body responds to an absence of the drug—sugar's hold over us is that powerful—but those cravings weaken over time as we consume less sugar.

As an interesting side note here: cancer tissues are warmer than the rest of the tissues in the body. When cancer feeds on sugar, it gives out heat. Expensive positron emission tomography (PET) scans that are widely used in cancer hospitals pick up on these heat signals. To do so, the patient gets injected with radiated sugar and the scan picks up where the sugar is concentrated—namely, where the cancer is! This also helps to explain why many have had success with sodium bicarbonate mixed with molasses or maple syrup, as it then works as a Trojan horse, getting the cancerous tissue to absorb the baking soda as it is "hidden" in the sweet molasses. I did not personally use molasses with my baking soda treatment, but it may work for you as many people have reported success with it. The standard protocol that seems to be most common is heating 1 part baking soda with 3 parts molasses or maple syrup in a sauce pan while stirring it. The suggested dose is then to take one teaspoonful three times daily for a month in between meals. (This would be instead of the baking soda in water protocol that I followed myself.)

Because cancer is warmer than normal tissue, there is a non-invasive and effective way of detecting these heat signals: thermography. Many people choose to use thermography instead of, for example, mammograms, as thermography is a harmless method but also detects cancer earlier than mammograms.

> **"Cancer cells demonstrate a three- to five-fold increase in glucose uptake compared to healthy cells."**
>
> *— Demetrakopoulus, GE*

17

It is believed that glucose released during times of stress not only feeds cancer but can even trigger it. This would explain why grieving a loved one, for example, or having other severe stressors in your life can trigger cancer. It rings true in my case, and I have noticed through the years that this is also the case for many other people diagnosed with cancer whom I've spoken to.

Another reason to avoid sugar in the diet is because the body needs vitamins and minerals to digest and process it, which could leave your body nutritionally deficient. It is so very important to provide the body with nutrients when you have cancer.. We'll talk more about this in the step that covers nutrition.

Diet sodas are just as bad as the sugar-laden ones—especially the ones containing aspartame, as aspartame is potentially carcinogenic. Cutting out all sodas, whether they are the diet kind or not, is important when working to restore your health.

Summary:

Sugar feeds cancer and is also the most acid-forming food you can consume.

Cut out as much sugar and as many sugary foods and drinks as you possibly can. Replace them with healthier options, such as stevia for sweetening and pure water and green or herbal teas for drinks.

Be mindful of foods that end with –ose, especially in the initial stages.

Glucose is believed to be one of the worst of sugars when one has cancer. Glucose is released in the body when you're stressed.

3

Oxygen

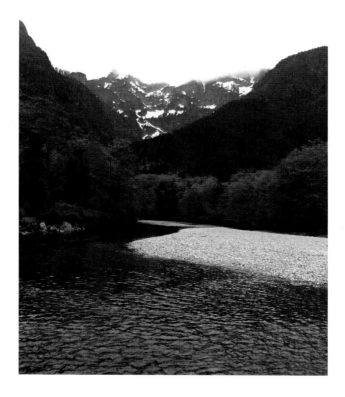

We all know that without oxygen, even for just a few minutes, we'll die. The methods I'm outlining here require oxygen's power to work; plenty of oxygen provision to the body is key. According to molecular biologist Dr. Stephen Levine, "In all serious disease states, we find a concomitant low-oxygen state. Low oxygen in the body tissues is a sure indicator for disease. Hypoxia, or lack of oxygen in the tissues, is the fundamental cause for all degenerative disease."

Further on in this book we will talk about how fresh, whole, non-GMO, sun-ripened, enzyme-rich, alkalizing, and plant-based foods restore oxygenation to the cells and help bring up pH levels. And let's repeat what Otto Warburg discovered: **cancer cells cannot survive in an alkaline and highly oxygenated environment.**

But another way of providing oxygen to the body and increasing pH levels is through exercise. While researching this book, I found that exercise lowers insulin levels, which creates a low-sugar environment that discourages the growth and spread of cancer cells.

You don't have to be an Olympic athlete to achieve good alkalinity through oxygenating your body with exercise. Moderate exercise like a brisk walk out in the fresh air can be very helpful, and as you get more exercise, you'll find you *want* more exercise—it's a great cycle.

If you are well enough to exercise, the ultimate is to exercise outside in the fresh air. However, that might not be possible for you. For a long time, I had a bad back and leg from an injury after a fall with a horse and wasn't able to exercise enough. What I could do was frequent deep breathing exercises that used my diaphragm.

This is how:

Sit with your back straight and your feet on the floor, a bit apart.

Breathe in through your nose with your mouth closed.

Fill the lower part of your stomach first, and then the upper part and your lungs on a count of four. Breathe out with your mouth opened as if you are fogging up a windowpane, also on a count of four.

These breathing exercises can be done anywhere, of course, but to maximize that flow of wonderful healing oxygen into your bloodstream, it's best to do this outside in the fresh air. I do these breathing exercises while out for my trail walks; the forest air is full of oxygen. I breathe in for four steps and out for four steps. When I was first starting my path to recovery, I would also visualize that I was breathing "into" the tumor, killing it with oxygen.

The fact that oxygen kills cancer is also one of the reasons why meditation is so beneficial: you bring in large amounts of oxygen while mindfully breathing, all while using good posture. Another reason meditation is helpful is because it is great at reducing stress. And again, when we are stressed, we release the stress hormone cortisol, as well as glucose, which is sugar—and as we've seen, sugar feeds cancer.

If you are going through traditional treatments and are very tired, it is advised to not overexert yourself—you need your rest to heal. This is where breathing exercises come in handy, too!

Side note: A wonderful tool I tried for a while was the ozone sauna. Apart from knowing that it helped my pH levels, I would feel energized and the skin smelled absolutely wonderful afterward, like I'd been out in the fresh winter wind all day. The ozone is taken up by the skin and is another way of providing the body with alkalizing oxygen.

Finally an observation made for yet another piece of the puzzle of why it's logical that there's a link between too little oxygen to the body and cancer. 60% of people with cancer are 65 or older. The risk for cancer in older age makes sense as the majority of people get less active and therefor gets less oxygen.

Summary:

Cancer cells cannot survive in an alkaline and highly oxygenated environment.

Exercise is a way of providing more oxygen to the body.

Deep breathing and walking outside in the fresh air are also ways of providing more oxygen to the body.

4

Hydration

Another important way of alkalizing the body is through hydration. Personally I have always struggled with staying properly hydrated.

There are many wonderful things to discover about the benefits of healthy water. Plenty of water between meals helps to flush out toxins and keeps the body hydrated. Unfortunately, clean water with a naturally high pH that is also high in minerals is getting harder and harder to come by. It just isn't possible for everyone to get that fresh, clean mineralized water that is so good for you anymore. So here are some little tricks to help. First, let the tap run for a minute before collecting the water you are drinking, as this helps to flush out metals such as copper that can sometimes accumulate in the pipes. Put your glass of tap water on the counter for a while to let some of the toxins such as chlorine evaporate a bit. Before drinking, squeeze a slice of lemon into your water and then put the whole slice with the rind still on it into the glass, since lemon has an alkalizing effect once it enters the body. Lemons also contain antioxidant compounds called limonoids that activate detoxifying enzymes.

Pure coconut water is also very hydrating, and it also contains electrolytes and potassium. My new favourite is maple water from the maple tree. It is very nutritious.

When it comes to bottled water, I would opt for Gerolsteiner or Evian, as they both have a high mineral content and high pH.

It is best, though, to avoid plastic bottles as much as possible; I'm glad that Evian is now also available in glass bottles. Most plastic bottles are made with a combination of plastics that contain a number of cancer-causing chemicals; perhaps the most dangerous among them is Bisphenol A, or BPA. This substance has been particularly linked to breast cancer as it contains xenoestrogen (mimics estrogen), and many countries have banned it from use in drinking water bottles or for food storage containers. Gerolsteiner comes in glass bottles and is a carbonated water that also has high sodium bicarbonate, magnesium, potassium, and calcium levels. These minerals are indispensable to human health. Every little bit counts!

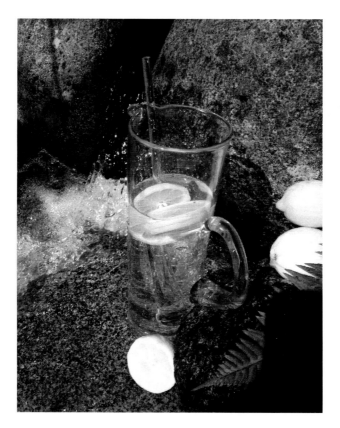

Not All Water Is Created Equal

Pure water has a neutral pH of 7. In certain areas of the world, one can find water that has a higher pH (because of its higher mineral content). An example of such a place is the Hunza Valley in Pakistan, home of the healthiest and oldest population in the world. The water in the Hunza Valley has one of the highest natural pH readings in the world. This water is also so highly ionized, mineralized, and pure that people in the region drink it straight from the glacial streams. Experts theorize that this is one of the contributing factors that allows the people in this area to be so healthy and to live so long. They also live simple, low-stress lifestyles while enjoying the outdoors and working the land. These people are reported to live to one of the highest average ages in the world and are apparently also able to bear children at an older age. In addition to their healthy lifestyles and healthy water, they also eat a diet consisting of organic, fresh, unprocessed, natural, and unadulterated food. One of these foods is apricots. They eat them fresh and dried, and even crack the pits open to eat the almond-shaped nuts inside. These nuts contain vitamin B17, also called laetrile, a method reportedly proven to be effective in fighting cancer and is also found in bitter almonds.

Acidic water doesn't hydrate the body properly, as is the reality of any fluid of a pH lower than 7. So you need to pay attention to the pH of the water you're drinking. If the water is acidic, those two recommended liters a day don't have the same hydrating properties as water with a neutral or alkaline pH.

Drink plenty of water away from meals (again, acids in your stomach are needed to digest the food and too much water dilutes them). I try to stick to green tea, herbal teas, coconut water, maple water, and, of course, plenty of the purest, healthiest water I can get.

I have read some conflicting information about water that has a very high pH, such in waters for example where the pH is forced and not natural. Again, the critique here is that it interferes with the stomach acids and alkalizes too much for too long, though some others say it's only beneficial. I say, follow your intuition and do everything in moderation. For me, it makes sense that aggressively alkaline water could be beneficial in the initial stages when you're trying to get on top of your pH levels, but that once a desired state has been achieved, opting for a "gentler" alkalinity in your water may be best.

In any case, water should, at the very least, be neutral or above on the pH scale.

I think that this explanation from Mihalovic, writing in *The New Agora,* sums up the connection of hydration and oxygen nicely: "Hydrogen ions tie up oxygen. That means that the more acid a liquid is, the less available the oxygen in it. Every normal cell in our body requires oxygen for life and to maintain optimum health. Cancer cells, on the other hand, need an acidic environment to grow."

To make this more understandable, think about acid rain. According to Mihalovic, "without going into a discussion of the chemistry involved, just understand that it's the same mechanism involved when acid rain 'kills' a lake. The fish literally suffocate to death because the acid in the lake 'binds up' all of the available oxygen. It's not that the oxygen has gone anywhere; it's just no longer available. Conversely, if you raise the pH of the lake (make it more alkaline), oxygen is now available and the lake comes back to life. Incidentally, it's worth noting that cancer is related to an acid environment (lack of oxygen)—the higher the pH (the more oxygen present in the cells of the body), the harder it is for cancer to thrive."

Summary:

Stay hydrated with pure water that has a pH of 7 or above.

Squeezing a lemon slice and putting it, rind and all, into a glass of water helps to alkalize it a bit.

5

Nutrition

Acidosis

People with a very low pH have acidic bodies, a condition called acidosis. This makes the body need to borrow minerals such as magnesium, calcium, sodium, and potassium from organs and bones to buffer that acid and remove it from the body.

As most people (if not all) with cancer have acidic bodies many natural health experts describe cancer as a *symptom* of acidosis— that cancer is a *symptom* of an unbalanced body environment. When one has cancer, it is therefore essential to replace those leached minerals and vitamins via diet and supplements.

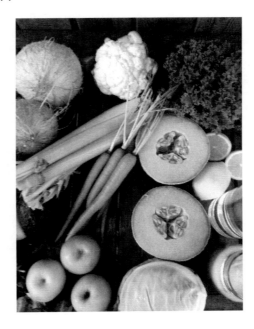

Alkaline Diet

Now, let's talk about one of the most challenging, but most transformational steps on the path to health: the pHood.

Before my cancer diagnosis, I had mostly seen food as food. Afterward, to my shock, I slowly started to understand that food is so much more than just fuel. I came to realize that maintaining one's health wasn't just about keeping the weight down, which mostly focused on how *much* food one ate, not so much about *what* one ate. I have never been really overweight and thought that as long as I kept my weight within the normal range, I could eat whatever I wanted. How wrong I was.

I started to understand that *what* one eats is where the focus should be. That food can not only be fuelling my body, but also *healing* it. That it can help keep the body strong and healthy and protect it from disease and illness. So instead of focusing on weight, you're better off focusing on nutrition. You might also find that while using these methods, your body finds its ideal weight naturally as one if its benefits is that it can balance hormones and reset the metabolism. I have also heard from people who have tried these methods, that not only do they feel and look better, but they've also found their right weight. The kind of foods and methods mentioned in this book are often also described as anti-aging. It just goes to show you that keeping things in balance yields results on many levels.

My holistic coach initially introduced me to the "Yin Diet," which I later discovered is in itself an alkalizing diet. After doing some research on alkalizing diets and finding that many people had achieved great success with them, I decided to stick to an alkaline diet as best I could. But it has been a bumpy road to get to where I am now, so hopefully I can make the path a bit smoother for you.

The mistakes and "don'ts"

One of the first "a-ha" moments I experienced after my introduction to an alkaline diet was how wrong I had been about things that I believed were healthy. I actually thought that, for the most part, I was already sticking to a healthy diet. For example, I made a smoothie every morning with ingredients that I thought were good for me, but soon after my diagnosis, I realized that they actually made my condition worse. What

I had thought was boosting my health was actually *feeding* the cancer. I was using orange juice and mangoes; although they contain vitamin C, these fruits were way too sweet for my condition. I was also including soy milk, and soy contains phytoestrogens that, I was told early on, imitate the human hormone estrogen; and that this is especially unwanted when you have breast cancer. (In addition to soy, yams also contain phytoestrogen). I have later read conflicting information on the subject of whether phytoestrogens are harmful or not, but nevertheless I stayed away from them. I also put flavored tofu into the smoothie—and again, since it is made of soy with additional sugar, preservatives, and food colouring, realized it should not have been a regular part of my diet. That smoothie also included yoghurt, and although it contains helpful probiotics, it is still advisable to stay away from it in the early stages of recovery, as it increases acidity for some and also mucus. There are several options for probiotics available in all health food stores and at naturopathic clinics. You can also try fermented foods such as sauerkraut which contain probiotics.

To make things worse, the yoghurt I was using was low-fat and flavored. Healthy fats help the body absorb necessary vitamins such as vitamin A, D, E, and K; eating nothing but low-fat foods can make it hard to process these nutrients. If you are low on these vitamins, it can impact your immunity and your body's ability to heal. I drank half a liter of this mixture—soy, OJ, mango, etc.—every morning and thought that I was being healthy, when in fact, every single ingredient was bad for me in my condition.

An important step in healing is to reduce the toxic burden on your body and cut back on acid-forming foods such as caffeine; nicotine; alcohol; sodas; milk; black tea; junk food like chips, sweets, ice cream, or desserts; processed foods; "fat-free" foods; and, of course, sugar. This is difficult for the first few weeks, but once your body starts to become more alkaline and has started to assimilate more nutrients, you'll notice fewer cravings for junk, or "empty," food. Just know that the cravings often get worse for a while before they get better. But rest assured, the craving for acid-forming foods will decrease and some cravings will disappear completely once you have balanced your body correctly. Apart from fluctuating cravings, another sign that your body is detoxing are the "die-off" symptoms. Some people report symptoms such as headaches and/or nausea when their body is detoxing the junk from years of toxic build-up. Personally, I got very tired when my body went through the first couple of weeks of detoxification, but I soon started feeling more energetic when my body got "cleaner." This is also common when going through a candida cleanse, which we'll discuss later.

I learned that a good template to follow for proper nutrition is to have 30 percent protein on your plate. The rest should be a combination of healthy vegetables. I opted for greens, sprouts, root vegetables, vegetables from the cabbage family, or brown rice, while sticking to berries for dessert. Don't worry that the protein might be acidic (as you might find in the chart provided further on) as long as it is a healthy protein because the body needs protein and also a little bit of acidity for digestion. Eggs, for example, are acidic but a good choice of protein as they are also rich in sulfuric compounds that help the body produce its own antioxidant, glutathione. The information on what foods are alkalizing or acidic vary a little bit. Potatoes are sometimes referred to as slightly acidic and sometimes slightly alkaline. I ate potatoes as if they were alkaline during my program and do occasionally still use them but sweet potatoes, which are indisputably alkaline, are my first choice.

(I try not to combine potatoes with chicken or turkey, as it's harder for our digestive systems to digest these if combined, as different enzymes are used and apparently this is even more prevalent if the potatoes are combined with red meats).

Now, don't panic. You don't have to go cold turkey forever on the things you enjoy. Just trust that every step toward a change will benefit you. You can try to exchange foods and swap them with healthier choices as you go along instead of going cold turkey. Lifestyle change takes time. It doesn't mean that you won't be able to enjoy the foods and drinks that you love from time to time once you have got on top of your pH balance and nutrition again.

Enzymes

What I found most challenging with my new alkalizing diet was that in the beginning, it was difficult to enjoy the foods I needed to be eating. My body wasn't really producing the healthy enzymes that are created in the mouth when we salivate. These enzymes are the body's first step in preparing our food for digestion. I suffered from stomach problems and therefore started taking supplement digestive enzymes for a little while (Wobenzyme). This made my digestion much better, helping me until I actually started to enjoy the new foods I was eating. It took time, but eventually I learned to make the food tastier and started to produce those enzymes without the help of supplements. Another thing that helped me reset my digestive system was not eating constantly, which gives the digestive system a rest and a chance to naturally reset.

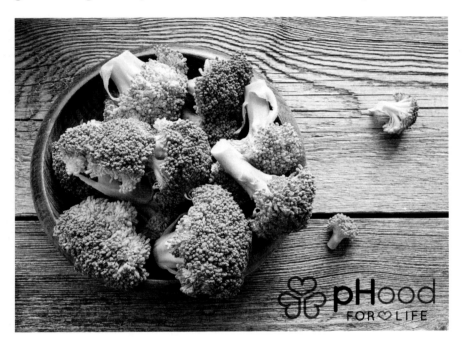

Better choices

The diet I started was rich in leafy greens and lots of vegetables from the cabbage family such as kale, broccoli, and green cabbage. Cruciferous vegetables like Brussels sprouts, cabbage, broccoli, and cauliflower are all high in fiber that promotes gut, kidney, and liver health. They also contain the phytochemical sulforaphane, which studies show helps to fight cancer.

I cut out all dairy except for butter (or ghee, a type of clarified butter) and cottage cheese. Butter is alkalizing and contains conjugated linoleic acid, which protects against cancer. On top of this, it also contains both vitamins A and D, which are good for immune function. These are not things we learn in school and I, for one, grew up thinking that margarine was better for me.

On my new diet, I stopped eating white rice completely and instead swapped in brown rice, sprouts, ancient grains such as quinoa, and occasionally potatoes (in particular, sweet potatoes are very alkalizing and also contain vitamin B6). Avocadoes became an almost daily staple in my diet for their alkalizing properties, high nutritional value and healthy fat.

I am a breakfast person and I found breakfast the most challenging meal on this new diet. I mostly stuck with oatmeal but tried to vary my morning meals the best I could. Oatmeal sprinkled with cinnamon or cardamom, and served with almond, rice, or coconut milk and dried dates is delicious and keeps me satisfied for hours. Oats are rich in soluble fiber that helps to promote a healthy gut and is still a staple in my diet. Since oatmeal is acidic I soaked it in apple cider vinegar first. More about this later in the book.

I would occasionally have grape fruit with coconut milk poured over it or an egg and a piece of yeast free manna bread or toasted sourdough bread (doesn't contain yeast) to vary things up. I sometimes had scrambled eggs with vegetables such as peppers or spinach. It was suggested to me to eat the left overs from my dinner for breakfast but that never worked on me. I found that when I figured out what resonated with me I was more likely to stick to it.

Red meat was exchanged for occasional poultry. I also included almonds or eggs for protein.

I would use lemon juice or apple cider vinegar with olive oil on my salads to make dressing. Apple cider vinegar boosts alkalinity in the body and also makes the skin soft and gives it a lovely sheen. Try to avoid low-fat or fat-free bottled dressings, as many of these contain large quantities of sugar.

Here are some tips on how you can upgrade poor diet choices with healthier ones, as certain foods are harder to go cold turkey on:

- Exchange potato chips for organic popcorn; sprinkle with minimally processed sea salt. A bit of butter is fine, as butter is alkalizing. But as popcorn is hard to digest, kale chips are an even better choice.

- Exchange alcohol, soda, juices, and coffee for water, coconut water, lemon water, green tea, herbal teas, and home-juiced veggies.
- If you still crave bacon, try to swap it with something else, even turkey bacon. Most bacon contains sugar and preservatives.
- Exchange pancakes for banana/egg pancakes (recipe below)
- Exchange regular table syrup for molasses or maple syrup. Bear in mind that none of these syrups are advisable if you are still in the process of beating a cancer diagnosis, as they are all a type of sugar, only a more nutritious choice.
- Exchange margarine for real butter.
- Coconut oil is great to fry in because of its high heat tolerance, but skip hydrogenated oils. Hydrogenation is a process that gives an oil a longer shelf life but produces fatty acids that inhibit the function of insulin receptors. So avoid cooking with products that are hydrogenated such as margarine for example. Coconut oil also has antifungal properties.
- Exchange sweets for berries (or the occasional piece of dark chocolate—chocolate over 70% cocoa has great antioxidant properties).
- Exchange red meats for "white" meats like pork or lean poultry, fish, beans, eggs, or almonds as sources of protein.
- Exchange cow's milk for goat's milk, unsweetened (or even homemade) almond milk, coconut milk, or unsweetened rice milk. Milk has lactic acid and is mucus-forming, and unless you opt for organic, it may contain growth hormones and antibiotics. (Mucus-forming foods are understood to being acid-forming in the human body). Or check out vegetable based milks as they typically contain more protein than, for example, store bought almond milk.
- Exchange aged cheeses for goat cheese and mozzarella. Avoid blue cheese in particular as it also contains mould.
- Exchange peanut butter with for pumpkin seed butter or, almond butter as these are the most alkalizing of the nut butters.

Above all, Think FRESH!

Some important notes on food in general:

I quickly learned that the more a food has been processed, the fewer nutrients it contains. The more food has been cooked, the fewer nutrients it contains. Lightly steamed vegetables typically contain more nutrients than if boiled. Fried foods contain fewer nutrients than if baked in the oven. Another thing to keep in mind is that frying or grilling meat at high temperatures releases "advanced glycation end products (AGEs)," which have been linked to cancer and put stress on the digestive and immune systems.

I stopped using microwaves once I realized how the food gets hot in a microwave —essentially, the food is irradiated with microwaves, a form of electromagnetic radiation that excites the molecules. Most natural health advocates warn against any food that has been heated with a microwave. The reasoning behind it is this: The cells that warm the food are actually water. They vibrate at such intense speeds that they break apart and are essentially deformed. If you've ever been introduced to Dr. Masaru Emoto's work with water, you'd understand why you wouldn't want to eat microwaved food. It responds to microwaves about the same way it responds to someone saying "I hate you" over and over again.

Needless to say, the less a food has been tampered with, the better it is for you. The more ripe it is before being picked, the more "ready" a fruit or vegetable is for your body to absorb its nutrients. So, the ultimate situation for that veggie, fruit, or berry is to not be tampered with; be cultivated without pesticides; non-GMO (genetically modified foods are, of course, the least natural of foods); not microwave-heated; and without added "flavors," fillers, or preservatives. All food you eat for ultimate nutrition should be ripe and ready to be harvested, then eaten immediately. The worst-case scenario involves eating highly processed foods that contain artificial colouring, various packaged food industry additives, and pesticides, and that have been genetically modified and then heated in a microwave and stored in plastic containers. If I need to heat up my food, I now always use the stovetop, toaster oven or the oven.

Though it's nearly impossible to eat perfectly in today's world, it is good to have an understanding of what direction to aim for when making choices from the options available. If you are savvy in the kitchen and have lots of time and money on your hands, there are plenty of yummy recipes you can use to cook great-tasting, nutritious foods. I suspect, though, that most of us don't have the luxury of time, or maybe even the necessary cooking skills, and benefit greatly from keeping it as simple as possible in the beginning. My advice is: experiment with your own combinations of these foods as you go along.

Another thing to realize is that some alkaline foods are more alkaline than others, while some acidic foods are more acid-forming than others. In other words, some foods bring the pH levels up more, and are therefore worth making a real effort to add to your diet. Remember that the goal is to have slightly alkaline blood—a little bit above 7. There's also a "grey zone," with some foods working alkaline in some bodies while causing others to be acidic. People who have a lesser ability to metabolize weak acids might need to focus on foods that are more alkaline. This might explain some of the mystery of hereditary cancers. I believe that I didn't necessarily inherit the gene for cancer from my mother, but that I perhaps inherited an inability to metabolize weak acids, and so my body became acidic more easily than someone whose body doesn't have that inability. I therefore need to be more vigilant about the alkalizing of my body than someone who has an easier time with breaking down acids. pHood for thought...

Now it's worth mentioning that even though a food may be less alkalizing than others—or even acidic, like tomatoes—that food may still be very nutritious and/or have anti-cancer effects. Once you've found your body's pH balance, you can consider reintroducing these nutritious options in moderation. The ratio recommended by some nutritional experts in a healthy body is 80 percent alkaline foods and 20 percent acidic. In a compromised body, such as after a cancer diagnosis, the recommended ratio is 90 percent alkaline and 10 percent acidic.

I went through a bit of a "grieving" process when adopting this new diet. I adored creamy sauces, steak, and a glass of wine. But interestingly enough, after a while, not only did the cravings dissipate, but my palate also changed. Now, creamy sauces feel "too heavy" and so does meat. I can feel the difference in my digestion. On the very odd occasion that I do have a glass of wine nowadays, it often tastes like vinegar to me. The taste buds also get more sensitive when you have been on a "cleaner" diet for a while. Sweet foods will taste sweeter and salty foods saltier.

This will mean that gradually, you will automatically (and naturally) want to reduce the amounts of sugar and salt in your food.

Diet also has a direct connection with our emotions and mood. Once you've addressed your diet, you will likely notice a difference in your mood; you may also find you are able to tackle situations that are affecting your emotions better.

Summary:

A body with a very low pH must borrow minerals from the body itself to buffer that acid and remove it. It's therefore important to replenish the body with vital nutrients when acidic.

The more processed a food is, the fewer nutrients it contains.

A good guide is: 30 percent protein on your plate, fill the rest with healthy vegetables, and make sure the food is predominantly alkalizing.

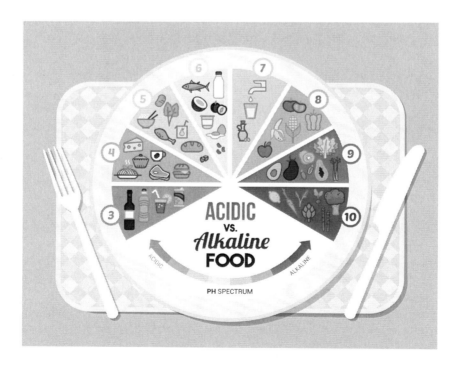

Most Alkaline Foods (the ones I personally use most often are highlighted)

Alfalfa
Almonds
Amaranth
Apples (Granny Smiths are not too sweet)
Apple cider vinegar
Apricots
Artichokes
Asparagus
Avocados
Bananas (ripe; but don't use too much as they can be mucus-forming)
Bean sprouts
Beets
Blackberries
Black olives (preserved in oil)
Brazil nuts
Broccoli
Brussels sprouts
Buckwheat
Butter/ghee
Cabbage, sauerkraut, and bok choi
Cantaloupe
Carob
Carrots
Cauliflower
Celery
Chestnuts
Chicory
Chives
Cottage cheese
Cucumber
Dates (dried)
Eggplants
Endive
Fennel
Figs
Flaxseed oil
Garlic (anti-inflammatory)
Ginger
Goat cheese

Goat milk
Grapefruit
Grapes
Green beans
Kale (contains vitamin A and more calcium than milk. See recipe for kale chips below)
Kelp
Kiwifruit
Leeks
Lemons
Limes
Lettuce
Mushrooms
Okra
Olive oil
Onions (contain fructo-oligosaccharides, a starch that nourishes friendly bacteria)
Papaya
Parsley
Parsnips
Pears
Peas
Peppers
Potatoes
Pumpkin
Quinoa (provides complete protein)
Radishes
Spinach
Stevia
Sweet potatoes
Watercress
Wheatgrass
Winter squash
Zucchini

Acid-Forming Foods—avoid these

Processed foods
Fried foods
Cold cuts
Condiments (such as mustard, ketchup, mayonnaise)

Seafood
Mature cheeses (the more mature, the more acidic)
Bacon
Margarine
Pastry
Ice cream
Bread
White sugar
Preserves
Meats
Pasta
Cereal flakes

Acid-Forming Drinks—avoid these

Alcohol (choose red wine if you do drink alcohol, as it at least has antioxidant properties; try to stick with the organic ones for less pesticides)
Coffee (acidic, but has antioxidant properties)
Black tea
Soda pop
Diet soda
Milkshakes
Commercially made fruit drinks
Cow's milk

Note: Soy and soy products are not acid-forming but are reported to create digestive problems and induce estrogen hormonal imbalances. Soy also contains glutamine which should be avoided, especially when fighting cancer.

Most Alkaline Drinks

Almond milk (make sure it's either home made or at least unsweetened as sugar is added in most of the store bought brands)
Herbal teas
Alkaline, pure, mineral water,

Acid Forming but healthy Vegetarian Foods

Cherries
Kidney Beans
Lentils
Plums
Pumpkin seeds
Rye
Sunflower seeds

Best Choices for Non-Vegetarian Protein (but acid forming)

Chicken (organic)
Eggs (organic)
Turkey (organic)
Buffalo/bison
Wild game (no antibiotics, growth hormones, or steroids and eat natural feed)
Fatty fish (such as salmon, sardines, haddock)
Grass-fed beef
Lamb

Examples of Foods/Herbs with Cancer-Fighting Properties

To my amazement, as I started this journey to health, I began to discover that nature itself provides us with an abundance of healing foods, drinks, and herbs. I had never seen food in this way before I started this journey. Now it's hard to imagine how blind I was to this reality.

Below are some foods, herbs and spices that are not all necessarily listed as alkalizing but which deserve an extra mention for their attributed healing properties or their nutritional value:

Artichokes (high in prebiotic inulin and help promote the formation of helpful bacteria in the large intestine)

Blueberries: This antioxidant berry is a staple in my diet. Blueberries have also been found to help protect against memory loss and prevent urinary tract infections.

Cardamom

Cayenne pepper

Chaga mushroom: This nutrient-rich fungus, which grows on birch trees, has amazing health-fortifying properties; many people with cancer have had great results with chaga. The chaga mushroom sucks nutrients from the tree; these nutrients are collected inside the fungus.

Cinnamon (helps to stabilize blood glucose)

Coconut (has antifungal properties)

Coconut water (very hydrating; contains electrolytes and potassium)

Essaic tea: Developed by the Canadian nurse Caisse from a formula she developed from First Nations (Native American) knowledge of healing herbs, this tea raises the body's pH and moderates blood sugar. She saved many cancer patients before she was shut down by Big Pharma greed.

Garlic: Garlic boosts the immune system, naturally reduces blood pressure, and is a natural antibiotic. It also enhances the production of hydrogen sulfide, which scientists believe helps prevent cancer from developing. It also stimulates liver enzymes that remove toxins from the body.

Ginger (a digestive tonic that aids circulation)

Green tea: I drink green tea daily. Yes, it contains caffeine, but it also has flavonoids, polyphenols that have anti-cancer properties. These polyphenols block the growth of blood vessels that support tumor growth and increase cell death in cancer cells. Green tea polyphenols also make cancer cells more sensitive to anti-cancer drugs.

Parsley (rich in antioxidants)

Pomegranate (rich in antioxidants)

Rosemary

Saffron

Shitake mushrooms (bolster immune function)

Turmeric (curcumin): Turmeric is attributed with killing cancer stem cells and is also said to make healthy cells stronger, whereas chemotherapy only kills the cancer's daughter cells while also compromising the immune system. More than 5,000 peer-reviewed biomedical studies have been published on turmeric. Turmeric is perfectly safe to use while undergoing chemotherapy and has anti-inflammatory and antioxidant properties. I try to use this amazing spice as much as possible (it's great in scrambled eggs, for instance). Turmeric is difficult for the body to absorb, so I try to use it as many ways I can. At the moment I am using a product that contains fulvic acid as it aids in the absorption of turmeric. You can also check out Dr. Mercola's recipes to help increase your turmeric uptake.

Check out the work of Dr. Russel Blaylock, M.D., to learn much more about the amazing cancer-killing properties of turmeric and the research that has been done on it. You do not want to miss out on the healing secrets of this spice.

Unrefined sea salt/Himalayan salt

Supplements and Oils

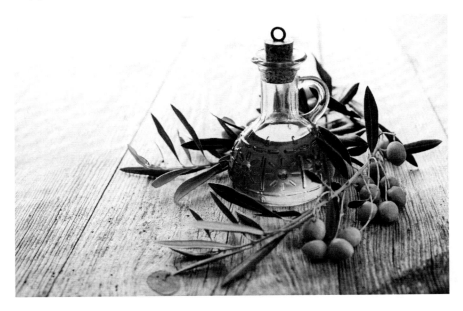

The soil today is highly depleted of nutrients and minerals, and in our modern society, we rarely get food that has been harvested when just ripened. As a result, we need to supplement our diet with additional nutrition. This is extra-important when fighting cancer, as essential nutrients are being leached from the body itself when one has cancer.

To boost my nutrition, I took a greens powder that contained most of the vitamins and minerals I needed to help replace the nutrients leached from my body and the greens also aided in balancing my pH as they are alkalizing.

The body needs healthy fats and oils to absorb nutrients. Healthy fats also line the cell membranes and help to lower blood glucose by making insulin more effective. Get the sugar connection here? Personally, I used oils and fats such as flax oil (which contains alpha lineoleic acid [ALA] and is one of the top sources of omega-3 fatty acids), olive oil, coconut oil, or butter with every meal in order to help absorb the nutrients I was eating. Primrose oil, borage oil, pumpkin seed oil (which also reduces your risk of stroke), coriander oil, sesame oil (which contains substances known to reduce cholesterol and prevent high blood pressure), hemp oil, avocado oil, and MCT oil are also all great healthy fats to consume. Be sure to choose cold-pressed oils; these preserve more healthful qualities through the extraction process. When using olive oil, I opt for an organic first cold-pressed brand, if available.

There has also been a connection made between cancer and vitamin D deficiency, particularly in people with breast cancer or prostate cancer. To help my vitamin D levels reach a healthy level again, I tried to follow the suggestion of spending 20 minutes in the sun without sunscreen and taking vitamin D drops during the winter months. Sunscreen not only blocks out the sun, which is the best source of vitamin D, but also often contain compounds that the skins absorbs and that can be harmful to the body.

It's important to understand that supplements are not to be used instead of good, healthy, nutritious food—they are to be used in addition to these foods. Vitamins and supplements are big business, but you certainly don't need to pay hundreds of dollars for good supplements. Start with a good alkalizing greens powder. I used Greens+ Multi, but there are several others that are just as good. I have a new favourite brand of greens powder that also contains the protein needed for one meal, which I put in my juice or in my smoothies.

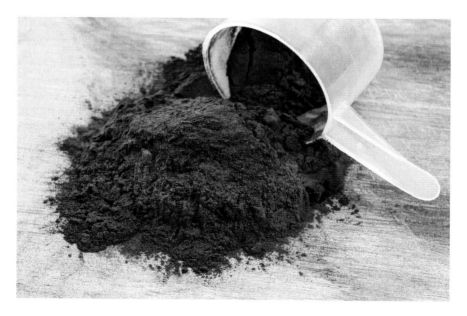

Apart from supplementing my body with sodium bicarbonate (initially) and a good greens powder with multivitamins, I also added iodine to my regimen. Iodine is a trace element that the body needs but doesn't produce on its own; it has been attributed with many health benefits, such as improving cognitive abilities, detoxing fluoride, improving metabolism, protecting the thyroid, balancing hormones, increasing energy levels, and protecting against pathogens and radiation. Most importantly, through a process called apoptosis, iodine has been claimed to help the body kill off cells that could end up leading to cancer. In addition, it's been suggested that it may help treat psoriasis. I took iodine drops every day for the first three months of my recovery and I suspect that my iodine intake was also one of the factors that helped me rid myself of psoriasis. In his book, *Sodium Bicarbonate, Nature's Unique First Aid Remedy*, Dr. Sircus states, "Sodium bicarbonate acts as a powerful, natural, and safe antifungal agent, which, when combined with iodine, covers the entire spectrum of microbial organisms (2)."

And, again but not surprisingly, iodine also aids in balancing the pH levels.

Another powerful tool against cancer is frankincense oil, as it promotes healthy cell regeneration and...wait for it...raises the pH levels. It is antifungal, anti-inflammatory, and antibacterial. Some claim that it is effective even against cancer cells that have been resistant to chemotherapy. I just recently tried this oil out, as it has many health benefits, and noticed that the "staying power" of the increased pH levels lasted a couple of hours. I have heard suggestions to put a drop of frankincense oil on the roof of the mouth every two hours when battling cancer. I tried this for a few days to see how my body would react and my stomach started hurting a bit. I increased my probiotics and was then fine. Now, I am not advising anyone to experiment like I do. I am simply sharing my experiences to help you make up your own mind regarding what you want to investigate further and what resonates with you. Of course, as with everything, even certain natural treatments may not be suitable for everybody and may have repercussions if taken to excess.

Summary:

Greens and healthy fats help to restore the nutrition leached from the body when one has cancer.

Iodine can be used to support thyroid function, among many other benefits.

Cancer patients are often deficient in vitamin D. The sun is the best source of vitamin D. Sitting in the sun without sunscreen for 20 minutes daily or taking vitamin D drops can help against vitamin D deficiency.

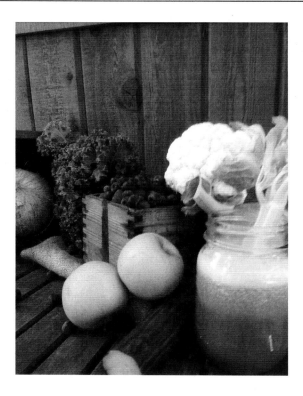

Juicing—the "Veggie Rush"

There's another important step in providing the body with nutrients: juicing. Drinking juiced organic vegetables and fruit not only provides the body with healthy nutrients, enzymes, and phytochemicals, but it also detoxes the body by neutralizing free radicals, strengthens the immune system, and reduces inflammation. It helps to reduce blood pressure, improves circulation, and increases energy. When you juice, you also give your digestive system a chance to rest and repair itself. Many cancer patients with stage 4 cancers claim to have actually cured themselves by juicing alone.

There are many juicers available today. Many nutrients in vegetables are concentrated just beneath the skin, so some juicers are probably better than others at extracting as much goodness as possible out of the veggies you use. However, I believe that any juicer will do—the key thing is that you're using it regularly. I used a very inexpensive juicer and solved the problem of making sure I got as much of the good stuff as possible by putting a tablespoon of the leftover pulp into my juice before drinking it. You can also add protein powder to your juices to make them even more nutritionally potent.

If you can't afford to buy a juicer, consider asking a friend if you can borrow one for a few months while you get on top of your health again.

Some people experience certain side effects to juicing that are worth mentioning. If you are juicing very frequently, you could experience tummy aches, diarrhea, and/or hemorrhoids. I got tummy aches, but was able to resolve the issue by listening to my body. I took a break from juicing for a while and then spaced my juicing sessions out until I figured out how my body tolerated it. I found that juicing one glass every three days worked best for me. You can also try diluting your juice with some water or chilled green or herbal tea.

I started juicing organic cucumber (contains B vitamins and detoxes your liver), cabbage, broccoli, green apples, blueberries, and blackberries once every three days. Some people have difficulty digesting raw foods and I myself have a very sensitive stomach. My body had a hard time breaking down the raw veggies whether they were juiced or simply eaten, so it just didn't tolerate daily juicing. But, again, if I spaced my juicing out to every third day, it worked great.

There is an amazing feeling of tingling or, as I call it, a "veggie rush," a few minutes after drinking the juice. It is really such a boost to one's wellbeing!

I eventually also started to make smoothies regularly—but this time, I didn't make the "nutritious" smoothies that contained ingredients that didn't truly support my body. Instead, I learned to make smoothies that really amplified my health. Mixing a good greens protein powder with berries and almond milk or coconut milk makes for a whole meal. I occasionally add banana, almond butter, or soaked chia seeds into my smoothies to make them more filling. This is an excellent choice for a quick but healthy lunch when you're pressed for time.

Juicing Recipes

The #1 Juice

This is the recipe I used for the first few months. I didn't like the taste in the beginning, but it gets better.

1 part green/white cabbage
2 parts green apple
3 parts cucumber
2 parts broccoli
1 part blueberries
1 part black berries

After a while, I started introducing other veggies and changed it up a bit with beetroot, fennel, pears, celery, carrots, etc. Be creative. Always try to use more veggies than fruit so that you aren't drinking too much fruit sugar.

Summer Mellow Yum

1 part strawberries
2 parts cantaloupe
2 parts cucumber
2 parts carrots

There are also other recipes that people have had success with, such as using only carrots or the Breuss juicing recipe.

The Breuss Recipe:

I have never tried the Breuss recipe, but mention it because the famed cancer doctor, Dr. Breuss, had a lot of success with his cancer patients using it so it's worth checking it out. He suggested juicing beetroot, carrot, celery and black radish juice. He also noted that people with liver cancer in particular should include potato in their juicing recipes. I would be sure to check this out properly before following this advice, as I have also heard that raw potatoes are questionable. Check out "The Breuss Cancer Cure" for more information.

Summary:

Juicing vegetables detoxes the body by neutralizing free radicals, strengthens the immune system, and reduces inflammation.

Juicing helps to reduce blood pressure, improves circulation, and increases energy.

Should you get tummy troubles, you can try spacing your juicing out a little bit. I only juiced once every three days and still could feel the benefits.

6

Going Organic

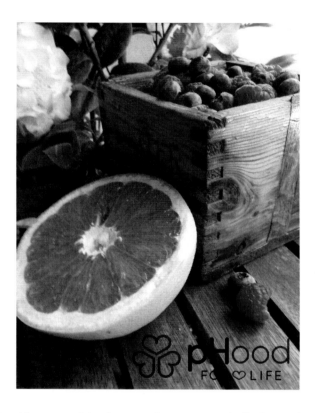

I was advised by a nutritionist to only use organic fruits and vegetables. In the past, I had thought that the hype was a little over the top and figured that if I just washed my veggies well enough to remove the pesticides, I would be fine. I soon discovered that there's much more to it than just pesticide residue. And, by the way, it's impossible to remove all of those pesticides because they are not just present on the surface; they become integrated into the plant from its soil and water uptake. My learning process in this area started with a suggestion from a prominent cancer doctor from Germany who recommended taking salvestrol as a supplement. A few days into taking it, I started to feel great, so I investigated salvestrol further and found out that it is a natural phytonutrient compound derived from organic foods only (found in many fruits, berries and most vegetables particularly the cruciferous ones). It isn't found in foods treated with pesticides. I learned that salvestrol production is nature's own way of protecting the plant from pests, fungus, bacteria, etc., and when we ingest this food, we get some of that protection for ourselves. The reason it isn't found in sprayed food is that plants sprayed with pesticides "don't need" the protection, so they don't produce it! I have since also learned that salvestrol further kills cancer cells in a process called aptosis in which the salvestrol is metabolized by the CY1B1 enzyme.

I was also advised to opt for organic protein such as eggs, meat, fish, and poultry to avoid hormones and antibiotics that could affect my already compromised immune system. Once I learned more about diet and health, that became a given for me.

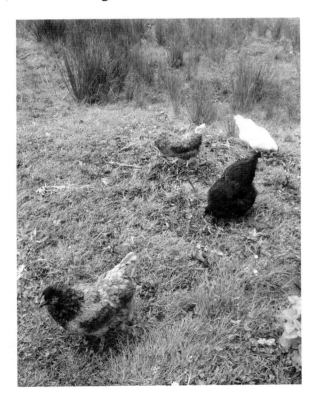

I also learned that there are other reasons for going organic: for instance, articles have suggested that organic eggs have much lower levels of salmonella compared to the eggs from mega-farm, caged hens (4.4% vs. 23%). According to Dr. Joe Marcola in an article on his website www. mercola.com, "Organic flocks are typically much smaller than the massive commercial flocks where bacteria flourish, which is part of the reason why eggs from truly organic, free-range chickens are *far* less likely to contain dangerous bacteria such as salmonella. Their nutrient content is also much higher than commercially raised eggs, which is most likely the result of the differences in diet between organic, free ranging, pastured hens and commercially farmed hens."

Organic foods are typically expensive and sometimes hard to find, so I understand if you have trouble fitting these into your diet. If you're using non-organic foods, make sure to wash them. I try to rinse produce in water with a couple of tablespoons of vinegar or a teaspoon of baking soda. This at least helps to reduce contamination. I find that carrots, cantaloupe, and pineapple are often more affordable in organic form compared to most other organic produce, as are avocados.

You can also look for organic produce on sale, or try shopping farmer's markets instead of large grocery stores. Sometimes you can find great deals on organic foods that cost way too much at pricey stores. Small local farms might not list their foods as organic, because that requires an expensive certification process, but may produce their crops using methods that meet or exceed organic standards—be sure to ask the farmer. You might also be able to get good deals by joining a Community Shared Agriculture (CSA) plan, where you pay up front and receive fresh food at a discounted rate, helping the farmer purchase seed and equipment.

If nothing else, try to avoid the foods listed below as part of the "Dirty Dozen" and purchase instead the "Clean Fifteen." The "Dirty Dozen" is a list of the foods that most commonly contain the most toxins if not produced organically. The "Clean Fifteen," in contrast, are the foods usually with the least toxins. The best thing to do, overall, is to eat a varied diet, rinse all produce, and choose organic whenever possible.

The Dirty Dozen

1. Apples
2. Celery
3. Cherry tomatoes
4. Cucumbers
5. Grapes
6. Hot peppers
7. Nectarines
8. Peaches
9. Potatoes
10. Spinach
11. Sweet bell peppers
12. Strawberries

Dirty Dozen Plus: Kale, collard greens and summer squash

<u>The Clean Fifteen</u>

1. Asparagus
2. Avocados
3. Cabbage
4. Cantaloupe
5. Sweet corn (beware of GMO, as corn is the #1 GMO crop. More on GMOs below.)
6. Eggplant
7. Grapefruit
8. Kiwi
9. Mango
10. Mushrooms
11. Onions
12. Papaya
13. Pineapple
14. Sweet peas (frozen)
15. Sweet Potatoes

Going GMO-Free

Many people are now aware that genetically modified foods exist, but if you haven't heard of them until now, allow me to briefly summarize what they are and why you want to avoid them. A GMO or GM food is one that has been genetically modified in a lab to contain certain traits that certain biotech companies and/or large industrial agriculture companies have patented. These traits are patented to enable the companies to earn a profit, *not* to "save the world from starvation" or "make farming more sustainable". Foods like corn, soy, wheat, rice, and other staple crops are often genetically modified to allow them to be sprayed with heavy doses of herbicides and pesticides without harming the plant. Ostensibly, this was intended to make growing them easier for farmers. Planting GMO seed was supposed to allow the crops farmers wanted to thrive, while weeds and pests were kept at bay. Before getting into the health hazards of the food grown with such biotechnology, you should know that GM crops did not thrive in the way that these large biotech and industrial agricultural companies promised. It is also important to note that the biotech industry, as represented by these companies, is intimately tied to the pharmaceutical industry. In fact, one of the largest pharmaceutical companies in the world was directly spun off one of these biotech companies.

The crops that these biotech companies spent billions developing have caused super-weeds and super-bugs, made us more resistant to antibiotics, and cross-pollinated with heirloom plants that took thousands of years to emerge. Many of these plants had their own natural, hardy resistance to bugs and weeds—the very qualities that biotech companies claim they were trying to create.

Biotech also failed to improve crop yields, meaning that a GM plant doused with these companies' profitmaking glyphosate herbicide— which has now been declared "probably carcinogenic" by the World Health Organization's cancer research arm—is no better at growing more plants or healthier plants than its conventional counterpart.

Then we get to the plants themselves. Biotech has spent money in similar ways to Big Pharma to cover up the cancer-causing traits of GM seeds. While farmers and gardeners have cultivated crossbred or hybrid plants for centuries, these plants did not have their DNA spliced and diced, or "edited," as they like to say now, to contain completely foreign genes. For example, GM corn, one of the most widely planted crops, was designed to contain a pesticide right inside the plant. That means instead of just spraying the chemicals onto crops, these plants are bred to contain them in their leaves, stems, petals, roots, and so on. This patented crop, actually contains a soil bacterium that produces insecticidal toxins which means that any time you eat this product, from the corn chips to high fructose corn syrup, you are ingesting these toxins—a pesticide meant to kill off pests. Unfortunately, there is ample evidence that eating pesticide, whether sprayed on or developed by Big Biotech to be inside the food, is extremely hazardous to your health.

To make it as obvious as possible that you should try to eat organic, non-GM foods, let's look at a controversial study performed by Eric Seralini and his peers. They examined a study submitted for a GM corn strain by one of the largest of the Biotech companies that stated that no adverse results were found after they fed rats this GM corn for 90 days. Seralini and his team found that this was not the case, and that there was evidence of liver and kidney toxicity which was glossed over. They decided to conduct their own study of rats fed GM corn, and what they found was so astonishing that the biotech industry tried everything it could to cover up the results—including trying to persuade the scientific journal that published the findings to retract the study from publication, which they did, only later to reprint the information after pressure from other concerned scientists who were studying adverse GMO effects.

So what did Seralini find? His rats, fed GM corn in the subsequent study, were riddled with tumors. There are now pictures all over the internet that show rats with lumps larger than their heads. Seralini found that GM corn was acutely toxic to the liver and kidneys of these animals, and that they were 100 percent more likely to develop cancerous tumors.

Other reports indicate that Big Biotech often restricts testing to a short of a period as possible so that studies end before cancer and other health hazards start to show up in the rats. Then, the company can say their product is safe because the rats didn't show any evidence of illness... (yet!). And if these hazards *do* show up within three months, the study is shut down so that it cannot be classified as a "proven study."

There have been many more studies on GM foods, but ultimately, the choice is up to you. Why would you want to eat something that is sprayed once, twice, sometimes *five* times with cancer-causing pesticides, herbicides, rodenticides, and other toxic chemicals before it is harvested? There are much cleaner, safer foods out there once you realize just how sinister the biotech corporations are, creating "food" that kills in the name of profit and market control. Many European countries have banned GMOs, but the European Union is slowly being infiltrated with new treaties, laws, and agreements to help the large corporations sneak their GMO crops into the political machinery there as well.

Crossbreeding has been done for thousands of years by breeding the best examples with each other, but now cellular invasion technology is being used, sometimes even to the extent of adding *animal* DNA to give certain plants a longer shelf life!

There is another alarming development with GMO farming and pesticides: it's killing bees. Some of these large corporations even use their bee-killing ways to their own advantage, trying to make themselves look good. For example, they may plant more flowers for the bees with the money obtained from customers buying their GMO bee-killing products. It's not a lack of flowers that's killing the bees.

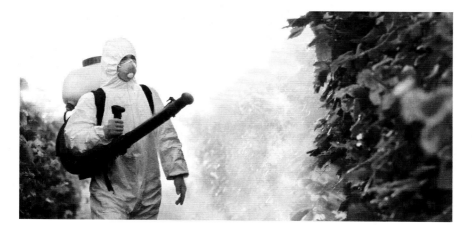

I have heard contradictory information about non-GMO and organic labeling. On one hand, some say that a food that is organic and carries an organic label isn't guaranteed to be non-GMO. Not even the farms that raise organic foods have an obligation to tell us whether their seeds are heirloom or GMO. But farms that raise their products organically are more likely to be ethical and more likely to feel the importance of raising non-GMO crops. On the other hand, some organic suppliers have told me that if a food is labeled certified organic, it is non-GMO. However, while this means genetically modified seeds have not been used, there still is a risk of cross-contamination; the biggest risk of cross-contamination is with corn crops, as their pollen is carried the furthest.

It may help to keep an eye out for the digits on the labels for fruits and veggies, as I have been told the following: organic always begins with a "9" and always contains five digits. Conventional fruit labels begin with a 4 and never a 9. And GMO products begin with an 8. If you live in Europe, you are better off, as GMOs are not permitted at the time I am writing this book—but that may change.

The profit-mongering of Big Biotech is a very difficult game to keep informed about, as these large corporations are also preventing the implementation of clear food labeling laws (though some states, such as Vermont, now have labeling requirements). So try to keep an eye out for products that *are* labeled as non-GMO and choose these whenever you can. When choosing non-GMO foods (even if all you can afford is a bunch of carrots), you not only prevent yourself from ingesting more dangerous foods, but also make a statement that you're *for* protecting the Earth.

Summary:

Organically raised foods are healthier for your body and for nature.

Pesticide-laden foods introduce toxins into the body and contain less protection for the body.

If using pesticide-sprayed veggies, try to opt for the "Clean Fifteen."

For a healthier choice, opt for foods labeled non-GMO when possible.

The Results

By now, you've traveled with me through the first part of my recovery journey: alkalizing the body, bringing it nutrition, hydrating it, detoxing it, and oxygenating it. So, what happened next?

Five weeks after my diagnosis, and still early into my alkalizing routine, my doctors did an MRI scan on my upper body to see if they could find any additional cancer. The results were read to me the first time I met the oncologist I was sent to see before my surgery because I didn't want to do radiation. At that time, it was discovered that the tumor had shrunk to almost half its original size in those few weeks. I had already noticed that the pain and feeling of blood being "drawn" to the area had dissipated after a few weeks on the baking soda, and that the skin over the tumor had got looser. Because I had been advised not to touch the lump since just after my diagnosis, this was the first time I had done so properly in several weeks. I clearly noticed how much smaller it felt; moreover, the lump had got a bit harder and felt as if it was "cut off" from the blood vessels and "contained" in a smaller shell. It now moved around much more easily, whereas it had felt "stuck" to my chest before. (This phenomenon, in which a tumor gets harder as it shrinks, has also been reported by others, but I haven't yet found a satisfactory description of the mechanics of why it would behave this way.)

I continued my alkalizing regimen up through to my surgery, which took place approximately eight weeks after diagnosis. When the pathology report from surgery came back, the tumor had shrunk about another 30 percent. So, all in all, the tumor had shrunk around 80 percent in just over eight weeks.

I was declared cancer-free.

At this point, I started to seriously research the natural methods that I had used and was shocked by what I found: **namely, the obvious connection between sugar and cancer, acidity and cancer, and toxicity and cancer.**

I encountered many medical texts, both from the natural health side of things and from conventional medicine, addressing the importance of acidity/alkalinity ratios and how they affect the body. However, I soon learned that some methods of alkalizing the body were being attacked by organizations that benefit from the cancer industry, such as pharmaceutical companies or "nonprofit" organizations that were bringing in big cash from donations for a "cure."

Online, there were thousands of entries and articles from people with a completely different view about the body and health, from former stage 4 cancer conquerors to former practitioners of traditional medicine turned natural health advocates. These often fit my very own experiences during the few weeks between diagnosis and being deemed cancer-free, and that I have continued to have to this day. These discoveries were shocking, but logical and liberating all at the same time.

Every day as I researched, I kept coming across more and more writings giving logical explanations of why the methods I was using were working for me. My aha-moments kept flooding as I eyed over sentences such as:

"The extracellular (interstitial) pH of solid tumors is significantly more acidic compared to normal tissues.

"Cancer tissues have a much higher concentration of toxic chemicals, pesticides, etc. than do healthy tissues."

"Alkaline foods and sodium bicarbonate are recommended so that the pH of the blood remains high, which in turn means that the blood is capable of carrying more oxygen."

"Toxins are not as easily transported out of an acidic body as in a slightly alkaline body. Cancer thrives in an acidic body."

With this type of information came epiphanies and, eventually, the big paradigm shift of understanding how the body works and how nutritious foods impact our bodies. I became obsessed with investigating this information and went through all of the emotions that follow such a realization, discovering a simple and logical explanation for something I had always believed was too complex to even try to understand.

But the learning process didn't end there. The next discovery was every bit as important as any other...

7

Gut Health

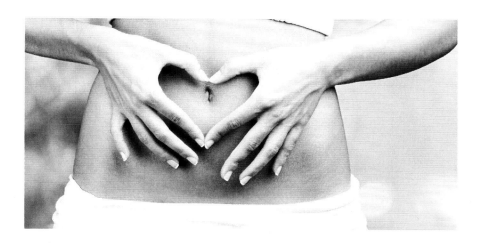

Follow your gut

If you've ever had a "gut feeling" about something, it likely wasn't just a whimsical intuition. Our guts are actually brilliant. They are, in fact, called our "second brain." Our guts and brains are interconnected via a vast circuitry of neurons that not only tell us when we need to eat, but also inform us of a million subtle things happening all around and in us. As I continued on my journey to reclaim my health and learned more about how to heal cancerous conditions in the body naturally, I quickly came to understand that a healthy gut is one of the cornerstones of overall health, and particularly in absorbing the nutrients the body needs to help fight cancer.

Antibiotics, among other things, can disturb the gut flora. I certainly found this to be true for myself. A diet high in sugar also disturbs gut flora, as does long-term unadulterated stress. Pesticides cause inflammation in the gut lining, and sugar is the number one factor behind leaky gut. Bad gut health can cause fatigue, joint pain, bloating, headaches, rosacea, acne, psoriasis, eczema, ADHD, and thyroid problems. Artificial sweeteners, antibiotics, exposure to pesticides and herbicides, and certain painkillers and birth control pills can cause yeast infections in the gut. The yeast strain called candida secretes toxins in the gut, and these mycotoxins eat the nutrients and minerals that we need while also releasing a type of alcohol that the body must constantly try to deal with. More about candida in a bit.

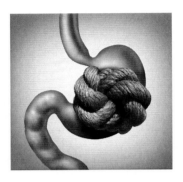

Fortunately, there are many different ways of promoting a healthy gut, such as:

- **Colon cleanses:** As Dr. Bernard Jensen puts it, "In the 50 years I've spent helping people overcome illness, disability, and disease, it has become crystal-clear that poor bowel management lies at the root of most people's health problems."
- **Healthy oils:** These help the body absorb more nutrients. I learned that the omega-3 to -6 ratio should be 2 to 1, since most people's diet is weighted too heavily with omega-6s. Poultry, eggs, avocado, and many nuts are among the foods that contain omega-6 fatty acids. Omega-3 fatty acids are found in flaxseed, walnuts, sardines, salmon, Brussels sprouts. This is a tough one for me, as I don't eat much fish at all but love avocado and eggs!
- **Enzymes:** Probiotics promote health within the lower gut and enzymes promote health via the stomach and higher up in the intestinal tract. You can find enzymes in the saliva, but they are also secreted by the pancreas, stomach, and small intestines in a healthy body. One of the reasons apple cider vinegar (ACV) with "the mother" (the active culture that makes it look cloudy) works so well is because it contains many of the enzymes that are missing from the modern diet. Without these enzymes, our bodies cannot properly break down food. Raw foods contain

the highest levels of these enzymes. I periodically still take the enzyme supplement Wobenzym N mentioned earlier.

- **Probiotics with healthy bacteria:** The healthy bacteria in your body make it more difficult for the "bad" bacteria, as well as viruses, fungus, and other harmful microorganisms, to take over. Fermented foods such as sauerkraut and kefir provide the gut with healthy probiotics, and you can purchase probiotic supplements online or in health food stores.
- **Overall nutrition:** Of course, eating a healthy diet overall, rich with easy-to-digest foods, helps gut health. As mentioned earlier, if you're not a vegetarian, eating broth made out of chicken feet, I've found, is great for the lining of the stomach, benefits muscle tissue and tendons, and also promotes collagen in the skin. Bone broth from beef bones also helps to promote good gut health.
- **Stress Release:** When stress activates the "flight or fight" response, digestion can shut down. The central nervous system shuts down blood flow, affects digestive muscles and decreases secretions needed for digestion. There are several ways one can decrease stress, tapping or EFT, for example. We will talk more about this later.

Getting a little personal, let's talk about poo. The following was news to me: in an ideal world, you should have a bowel movement two to three times a day (depending on how often you eat), preferably between 30 and 60 minutes after finishing a meal as this is indicative of a healthy digestive system.

When food sits in the intestinal tract for too long, it starts to rot. While we want food to break down so that our bodies can absorb the nutrients it can provide, we also want it to eliminate the stuff we don't need as quickly as possible.

This is also why it is so important to drink plenty of pure, fresh water in between meals. Being hydrated keeps the "flow" going through the bowels so that you can properly eliminate. For these reasons, the steps outlined in this book also helps to promote digestive health and regular elimination of toxins in the body.

Summary:

A healthy gut is better equipped to process food and absorb nutrients.

Healthy oils, enzymes and probiotics all help the gut to stay healthy.

Staying regular is important for detoxification.

Candida

Dealing with a candida overgrowth problem is also part of achieving good health in the gut and is essential for staying healthy. After following my alkalizing regimen, I was rid of the cancer, but a couple of months after my surgery, it was discovered that I had a candida overgrowth.

Candida albicans is a yeast that we all have in our bodies; it mostly resides in our gut. It does have a purpose at normal levels, but when there's an overgrowth of this yeast—most commonly after antibiotic treatments— it starts to cause problems. Healthy bacteria feeds on candida, but when the levels of good bacteria in the gut are altered, the candida sometimes grows out of control and can eventually turn into a fungus. This is why it is so important to supply the body with healthy bacteria, particularly after a course of antibiotics.

Once the candida yeast is growing strong, it begins to create mycotoxins. These mycotoxins permeate the blood and the lymph system, especially affecting the white blood cells and killer cells that are responsible for finding foreign viruses and bacteria and eradicating them. At this point, the immune system becomes depleted and eventually cannot fight the overgrowth of candida. The liver, kidneys, and other organs of detoxification start to run poorly and you have a perfect environment for cancerous cells to grow.

And cancer, it is believed by some, is one of the health problems inextricably linked with candida. My mother suffered from a candida overgrowth before passing away from cancer and since I, too, had both problems, I obviously take these theories very seriously. Whether or not there is a real link between the two, at the very least, they both thrive in the same conditions: a low-oxygen environment with a plentiful supply of sugar.

Candida, is so common a problem that some call it an epidemic. A Rice University study found that up to 70 percent of the population has a candida overgrowth. The good news is that it can be eradicated with natural treatments and lifestyle changes.

A myriad of symptoms are related to a candida overgrowth and many people suffer for years without recognizing the cause of the problem. Because of the number of symptoms and the difficulty in diagnosing candidiasis (the formal name for candida overgrowth), the problems can cause many trips to the doctor, often resulting in a diagnosis of hypochondria. For instance, the doctor of a friend of mine in my home country of Sweden refused her a candida blood test when she asked for it, despite not being able to diagnose her condition, which showed many signs of possible candida overgrowth. A simple test could have helped her find a solution or at the very least, rule candida out as a possible cause.

With help from my story, my friend was able to get rid of her overgrowth herself through diet and candida-fighting natural treatments and her issues were resolved. Debilitating issues she'd had for years were resolved in just a couple of months. With conditions like these I strongly recommend visiting a natural health practitioner for a second opinion as they are typically much more experienced with issues like overgrowth and how to treat it than your typical conventional practitioner.

Allergies, depression, brain fog, fatigue, painful joints, sinus congestion, weight gain, mood swings, abdominal pain, and cravings for sugar and alcohol are only a fraction of the many possible symptoms of candidiasis. There are also several different causes of candida. Among these are:

- Antibiotics killing too many of your friendly bacteria. When you take antibiotics, they don't just kill the bacteria you don't want in your body: they also reduce the good bacteria.
- A diet high in sugar
- Certain medications
- Stress

My gut was a mess from all of the antibiotics I had taken prior to my diagnosis. I was hospitalized in 2003 for Pseudomembranous colitis, a condition that can arise from taking certain antibiotics, and my stomach hadn't been the same since. The diet that was suggested to me at the time involved eating only bananas, white rice, and white bread. Knowing now what I didn't know then, I can see that this diet, prescribed by my doctor, is what eventually sent me to the emergency room. I also lived a very high-stress lifestyle.

Candida Symptoms

The symptoms one can get from candida are many and vary from person to person. I followed a scorecard after my diagnosis of candida overgrowth and during my recovery that listed some of the more than 50 possible symptoms. I was asked to score each listed symptom from 0–10, indicating the severity of the symptom, and then followed the suggested instruction on how to treat it depending on whether the score was mild, moderate, or severe. I scored as a severe case, just as the blood test had showed. About half of my symptoms scored a 0, but the other half scored much higher, especially on symptoms such as fatigue, headaches, and muscle weakness. Once I started the treatment, I went back to the scorecard each week and tallied up my numbers again to track my progress.

Here are only some of the symptoms that can be connected to a candida overgrowth and that were also included on the scorecard:

- Abdominal pain
- Anxiety or tearfulness
- Burning/tearing of eyes
- Chronic sore throat
- Confusion
- Constipation
- Cough or recurrent bronchitis
- Cravings for alcohol
- Cravings for bread
- Cravings for sweets
- Diarrhea
- Difficulty with decision making
- Endometriosis or infertility

- Eczema
- Fatigue
- Frequent colds and flu
- Frequent indigestion
- Headaches
- Heartburn
- Hives
- Impotence
- Inability to concentrate
- Insomnia
- Itchy ears/nose
- Irritability
- Loss of balance
- Low libido
- Menstrual irregularities
- Mood swings
- Mucus in stools
- Multiple food sensitivities
- Muscle aches
- Muscle weakness
- Nasal/sinus congestion
- Numbness, burning pain, or tightness in chest
- PMS
- Poor coordination
- Poor memory
- Poor sense of direction
- Postnasal drip
- Prostatitis
- Rashes or psoriasis
- Recurrent ear infections
- Sensitivity to foods leavened with yeast
- Sensitivity to mould
- Sensitivity to perfume, paints, or chemicals
- Sensitivity to tobacco smoke
- Shaking or irritable when hungry
- Spacey feeling
- Strong body odour
- Swollen or painful joints
- Thrush in mouth
- Vaginal infections
- White coating on tongue

Enough to make you go: Geeeeeze, stop already!

Now, should you have any or even several of these symptoms, it doesn't by any means indicate that you have a candida overgrowth. There can be several different reasons for these symptoms other than candida; several can also occur when you are too acidic, or for a variety of other reasons. It's also important to point out that having candida does not automatically mean that you have cancer. In fact, most people with candida do *not* have cancer. But should you have excess candida, it does mean that your gut is not in balance and you will feel much better if you get rid of the overgrowth of candida in it.

You can test for candida overgrowth through a blood, stool, or urine test.

Candida Treatments

Once it was discovered that I had candidiasis, I went on a very strict anti-candida diet for five months and used a natural treatment kit to help kill it off. The kit included caproil to kill off the candida (caproil is also found in coconut oil), psyllium fibre to "scrape" the inside of my intestines clean, and bentonite clay to help soak up the now-dead candida. The anti-candida diet resembles the alkaline diet but is much stricter.

I have since learned that raw vegetables are hard on the "candida-overloaded" stomach. So one of the challenges here is to cook healthy vegetables that are not too starchy in the beginning of the program. Ground flax seeds, pumpkin seeds, and chia seeds are good to include in the candida-fighting diet, as they apparently help force candida to revert from its fungal state into yeast again. There are other theories about candida and the difference between the fungal form and the yeast form but the information I am sharing here is from what I found in my research of it.

There are other products out there that help fight candida, such as colloidal silver, GSE oil, oregano oil, and the herb *Gymnema sylvestre*. I have discovered that it's best to include at least a couple of different candida-killing products in the program so that the candida doesn't grow resistant, which it might if you rely on just one.

During treatment and also after your candida growth is brought down to a healthy level, you should reintroduce friendly bacteria to the gut by taking probiotics on a regular basis. I usually take probiotics for three months and then take a three-month break to let my body rest and restore the bacteria naturally. I also rotate the probiotics I use to make sure my gut gets as many different kinds of healthy bacteria as possible. One of my favourite products is the Proalive Probiotic from Ascended Health; every batch is different so the body never gets "used" to the bacteria. We all have different bodies with different possible deficiencies and our bodies will respond differently to different good bacteria. It took me a while to find what worked best for me and what felt best for my stomach. The thing to remember is to try not to get overwhelmed.

If you do a candida cleanse, be aware that it's common to go through a "die-off" period when certain symptoms get worse for a short period before they get better. What's happening is that the candida is craving the bad things that feed it, and of which you are now depriving it. When the candida fungus gets killed off, it leaves little perforations in the intestines; as a result, food particles can get distributed out in the bloodstream more easily, sometimes causing temporary food allergies and sensitivities. This can cause different symptoms in different people, though a common one is itchy skin. When the intestines heal, the allergies normally go away. Of course, should you experience this, use caution to make sure that your symptoms are not for different reasons.

I have read several articles from natural health professionals stating that not only is an overgrowth of candida often missed by doctors or misdiagnosed, but antibiotics are often prescribed to kill it off when it is diagnosed correctly. What they all seem to conclude is that antibiotics are necessary, but these are really only a temporary solution. Oftentimes, antibiotic use just makes the situation worse in the long term as even more good bacteria is killed off in the gut by these over-prescribed drugs.

Candida and cancer connection?

Earlier in this book, we talked about the effects of baking soda on cancer. Sodium bicarbonate is used in emergency medicine and is also sometimes injected into a patient before administering chemo drugs as a way to protect the kidneys. But its uses against cancer itself are not accepted by conventional medicine. Conventional doctors that try sodium bicarbonate therapy for their patients often run into trouble. Some are stripped of their licenses and others are even sent to jail.

Dr. Tullio Simoncini is an Italian traditional oncologist who pioneered sodium bicarbonate therapy as a means to treat cancer. He realized early on that the conventional therapies against cancer were not working. "People were dying," he said.

Simoncini's theory is that cancer is a response to the fungal state of candida growth, and that sodium bicarbonate works as a fungicide to eradicate candida infections when injected. When I went to Rome to interview him, he told me the story of one of the first patients he treated: an 11-year-old boy who was suffering from lymphoma in the brain and who had been in a coma for two weeks. The boy's mother knew he was dying but she wanted to at least talk to him one more time before he died. The boy arrived at Simonici's ward in the morning; after having been intravenously treated with a large dose of sodium bicarbonate and nutrients during the day, the boy awoke and spoke with his mother. Dr. Simoncini was banned from medicine when it was discovered that he was using sodium bicarbonate in his treatments.

Very few agree with Simoncini on his theories of that cancer is the fungal state of candida, and from what I've learnt neither do I, but regardless of whether this is the case, both conditions respond to a sodium bicarbonate treatment.

Sodium bicarbonate treatment for tumors worked on me, and it has worked on thousands of patients, regardless of whether injected by a physician or self-administered and whether the underlying cause is indeed candida or instead an acidic body. Personally, I feel it is enough to have a solution to both "problems" or "symptoms," but in looking at an explanation, I am more inclined to follow the notion that cancer and candida are two separate issues that both thrive in a similar environment in the body and both feed on sugar. This is because even after I was declared cancer-free, I still was diagnosed with candida a few months later, and by that point, I must have had the condition for years. Moreover, Dr. Simoncini's only explanation for why I had success with taking sodium bicarbonate orally, rather than injected by a physician, was that I didn't even have cancer in the first place. This didn't sit right with me, as mammogram images, ultrasound, MRI, and 13 core samples of a biopsy helped diagnose an invasive cancer.

Ultimately, Dr. Simonici, who is still a staunch conventional doctor, and I basically only agreed on one thing during our interview, but that is okay, because that "thing" was that **sodium bicarbonate works on cancer** and we have both experienced its successes with treating cancer, albeit in very different ways. For me, this is enough for now.

The diet for candida sufferers is challenging because it is even more rigid as far as sugar goes. In the section for alkaline pHood ideas later in this book, some recipes and ideas are good for candida sufferers as well; they're all clearly marked. In my next book, which will be a cookbook with anti-cancer recipes, I plan to also include candida-friendly recipes.

The good news is that should you have to go through the challenge of ridding yourself of candida through diet and do it successfully, you will have graduated the "Anti Cancer Diet College." The anti-candida diet teaches you from the ground up what to focus on for a low-sugar diet, and helps you really enjoy the foods required to stay healthy. Eventually, once your body is back in balance, you can start to slowly reintroduce some additional foods that aren't on the plan into your diet. However, you may find that you no longer crave them at all!

Candida and iron levels

While researching candida, I came across interesting information that fungal candida "steals" iron from red blood cells. Iron provides hemoglobin, which is the part of your red blood cells that carries oxygen to all the cells in your body. This helps to support my own thoughts on why candida often is found in a body that has cancer: it has helped to deprive the body of oxygen. Interestingly, I was also iron deficient before my diagnosis (as many cancer patients reportedly are). Hmmm!

Even after being rid of candida for some time, I still struggled with my iron levels. I have since learned that the body needs B vitamins to help with iron uptake. B vitamins are found in foods such as meat, fish, dairy, poultry, and eggs. Since I almost never eat meat, fish, or dairy, I have had a hard time getting enough B vitamins. I have therefore started to augment the B vitamins I get from eggs and chicken with B vitamin supplements and my iron deficiency has been solved. Trial and error.

Summary:

Candida yeast fills a function at normal levels, but when there's an overgrowth, most commonly after antibiotics treatments, it will start to cause problems.

Because of the number of symptoms and the difficulty in diagnosing candidiasis, the problems can cause many trips to the doctor, often resulting in a diagnosis of hypochondria.

A candida cleanse and a strict candida diet usually take care of the problem, helped along by some good probiotics.

Candida overgrowth has been shown to have connections to cancer. The jury is still out on what these connections are, but there are reports that they both respond to a low-sugar diet and to sodium bicarbonate.

8

Cause?

Let's re-visit Otto Warburg's quote: **"Cancer, above all other diseases, has countless secondary causes. But even for cancer, there is only one prime cause, summarized in a few words: the prime cause of cancer is the replacement of the respiration of oxygen in normal cells by a fermentation of sugar."**

Knowing this and having addressed it, it's time to address the secondary causes and triggers. Most of us know the obvious contributing factors to cancer, such as the connection between smoking and lung cancer and between hormones and cancers of the reproductive organs. Obvious things that would help in these cases are to stop smoking or stop taking hormones such as birth control pills. But knowing now that there are many different contributing factors to cancer, one needs to take a closer look at one's own unique case. As with any illness, there is very seldom a "one size fits all" treatment for cancer. These methods are general and we are all unique people with different health histories. To get the best results, you need to get involved in your own situation and do some searching.

Once I was on track with pH balance, getting the right nutrition, boosting my gut health, drinking plenty of water, and providing my body with more oxygen, I started to look deeper into what causes cancer and the reasons for my particular case. This was an important step, because if I didn't try to eliminate the causes, triggers, and environment that made cancer thrive to the best of my ability, it would most likely return.

Because overuse of antibiotics causes problems in the gut, I am inclined to think that this was the main cause of my cancer, although not the only cause or trigger. For example, I was in a very stressed state during the years leading up to the lump starting to grow: I was overworked and got little sleep, got very little exercise, and unknowingly ate the wrong foods, among many other things which contribute to ill health. Little by little, you have to whittle these things down and deal with them if you want to improve your health. My suggestion to you is to try to figure

71

out what may have contributed to your particular illness. Do research, and if you are one of the lucky ones who has access to a good holistic or naturopathic doctor, pay them a visit to get their view on things and see if it resonates with you.

While it is crucial to address the physical causes of illness, the same goes for the different emotional stresses in life, such as great losses, grief, relationship issues, workplace dynamics, family issues, worry, etc. Bad stress produces hormones and glucose (sugar) that are detrimental to our health and which promote cancer. Through my journey, I came to understand that it is important to address these issues, heal, and then rid oneself of past traumas.

Setting boundaries is important, but we must also learn to forgive and forget (and that can also include oneself). I am a very different person from who I was before my journey with cancer and I am constantly changing—hopefully improving—and the greatest gift of all is what my journey with cancer has done for my fear. I am not scared of cancer because I beat it once and now understand the "secret" of it.As a matter of fact, I have very little fear of *anything* anymore. Once one has faced possible death, everything else changes, too. This doesn't mean that the cancer will never return, but the fear surrounding it has been dealt with. Of course, the usual worries still occur occasionally, such as with loved ones, finances, changes in circumstances, and so on, but these worries are of a different nature and pass more quickly.

Knowing that lifestyle and diet can so dramatically impact one's health and knowing one can help the organs along to fulfill their purpose, I wish that people would think twice before removing or compromising body parts, especially in a "preventative" fashion.

Remember that these organs do fill a function. The lungs help bring oxygen to the body. The thyroid helps regulate metabolism and has many other functions. The lymph glands help get rid of toxins in the body. (They took three of mine out, and now my body has to find other ways to do their jobs.) Breasts and ovaries fill functions other than in the reproductive stages of life; they play a part in the endocrine system in the post-menopausal stages as well. The road to health will be much smoother in a less compromised body.

There are many ways in which one can try to protect oneself from toxins that cause cancer. There are many wonderful herbs and products that help to clean and support the body against disease. There are more than 400 alternative methods that have been successfully used against cancer and that will also help to prevent it.

What you choose needs to feel right for you and resonate with you and your body. Listen and take in the information your doctors give you and go for second opinions if you don't feel confident that what they prescribe is right for you. Remember, *you* are in charge of your own body. *You* are the one who should make the informed decisions.

Summary:

"Cancer, above all other diseases, has countless secondary causes. But even for cancer there is only one prime cause, summarized in a few words: the prime cause for cancer is the replacement of the respiration of oxygen in normal cells by a fermentation of sugar."

As we all have unique health histories and situations, we need to figure out the causes or triggers for our own individual case.

By addressing cancer triggers, we can better protect ourselves from disease.

9

Stress Release

I already knew that stress is one of the biggest friends of cancer, but how it translated physically was still a bit of a mystery to me. As I came to realize that the body releases stress hormones and glucose in response to a "fight or flight" instinct, it all made sense. Glucose is sugar and sugar feeds cancer. As I kept testing my pH and learned how my body reacted to different circumstances, I began to understand why stress is the biggest enemy of a healthy body. The day after an argument or a stress session about finances for example, I noticed that my pH went down considerably despite making no change to my diet. I soon realized that relaxation methods were beneficial not only because one breathes better when relaxed with a supple stomach, therefore getting more alkalizing oxygen into the blood, but relaxation also helps with stress levels and decreases the glucose being fed to the cancer. Stress release activities help turn off the stress hormones adrenaline and cortisol. In my research, I found numerous articles on how reducing cortisol benefits the body when healing from cancer.

When going through any kind of stress, physical and emotional rest is imperative (and I can't think of many stresses worse than what a cancer diagnosis brings). I am not just talking about a healing "good night's sleep," but also taking a breather for yourself. Take a moment to relax. Ask friends and family to help out. You don't have to do it all yourself. Getting sick is a sign that your body and mind need a change. And your friends and family will often be glad to know that they can do something to help. Learn to set boundaries, ask for help and accept help. Remember: "Those who mind don't matter and those who matter don't mind."

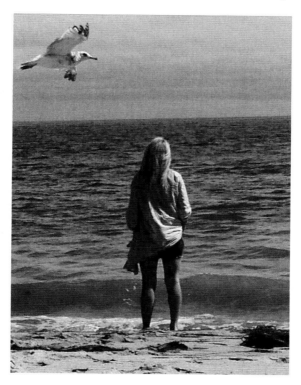

Relaxing and dealing with the body's "fight or flight" response when stressed doesn't necessarily mean you should go and lay on the couch. It could mean actually using the "fight or flight" response to deal with the chemical releases in the body. That is, you may consider taking these instinctive reactions and acting on them, using the muscles when the body is screaming to fight or flee; this helps to deal with these substances in a natural way. The theory is, being unable to physically act on this response in the body is when problems can arise. This also ties in with situations like stagnation or being in a stressful relationship. Sometimes we can be lonelier while in a relationship than when we're not in one. And long-term stagnation such as feeling "stuck" in a situation, be it a bad relationship or unemployment, can also contribute to high stress levels. Suppressing the emotions this causes is unhealthy. Sometimes getting ill is the body's way of saying no if we get in these situations.

Finding time to exercise is a challenge for many people, but even just a couple of minutes can have beneficial effects. As little as two minutes of doing squats supplies a surge of neurotransmitters, such as dopamine and serotonin (the same neurotransmitters targeted by antidepressants).

Addressing past traumas is a key ingredient in reducing stress. Many people don't realize that these traumas actually get stored in the body. The same way a librarian puts a book away on a shelf, maybe marked "death of a loved one" or "divorce" or "huge fight with my in-laws," the body takes an inventory of stress that it can't quite handle fully when it occurs and stores it away to take out and digest more fully at a later date. Sometimes cancer—or other conditions—is simply the body bringing our attention to an old trauma that hasn't been "fully read" and dealt with appropriately.

On my journey to recovery, I came to realize that one can never dismiss pain, grief, anger, sadness, etc. They must be fully felt and dealt with, not ignored, or they will come back to haunt you. That includes clearing up unresolved issues with people and situations in our life if they are causing us pain. Should you not be able to resolve trauma with someone who is causing or ignoring your pain, you may find it helpful to talk to someone you trust or a therapist that can offer you tools of how to deal with the situation or person. In some situations you may be better off to say goodbye and walk away from the toxic situation, relationship or "friendship", if possible, as it can cause sickness. I believe that finding healthy ways of dealing with traumas is absolutely vital to restoring and maintaining prolonged health and keeping cancer at bay.

Loss is a major stress factor and loss pertains to more than the loss of a loved one, a relationship or a job. Loss can be related to many different things, for example children leaving the family home, having to re-locate and leaving friends and familiar grounds, losing the ability to enjoy a hobby or losing the ability to exercise. When life is handing you too much to deal with, it can help to force your body and mind to slow down; for instance, you might physically move slower in certain situations or focus only on the task at hand. For example, when taking a shower, focus on the water and how it feels. When doing the dishes, move slower and focus on what you are doing, not thinking about anything else. Take a rest from your thoughts and just feel the moment. It's a little mini-meditation. This is why play is so therapeutic. You are in the moment.

A Word about Sleeplessness

As mentioned earlier, many newly diagnosed people experience a few months of insomnia. This is normal and there are many ways to try to relax, but know that after a while, all that waking up in the middle of the night usually disappears. If you do wake up in the middle of the night, try using the breathing exercises I mentioned in the section about "Oxygen" earlier in the book while lying down.

For stress release, you can also spend time in nature, meditate, paint, draw, write in a journal, relax in a bath with some lavender oil, watch a film that makes you laugh, or just have a good cry and let it all out.

Anything that releases stress and makes you calmer and happier will help stop feeding the cancer. Laughter is one of the most amazing tools for healing; don't overlook it!

Before my surgery I watched my favourite Monty Python films over and over again to try and make myself laugh. Inspirational books and movies can also help you calm down and gain perspective. The mountain climbing documentary *Touching the Void* tells a story of overcoming challenges and surviving against all odds. Watching this helped me tackle things one moment at a time, as seeing my situation as a whole was too overwhelming at times. Something as simple as watching Laird Hamilton surfing gave me yet another perspective on life and helped me "ride the wave of my life." Whatever helps take you out of your head and the tricky situation you might be in, even if just for a moment, helps to relieve the stress.

Here are ways that you might try to relieve stress.

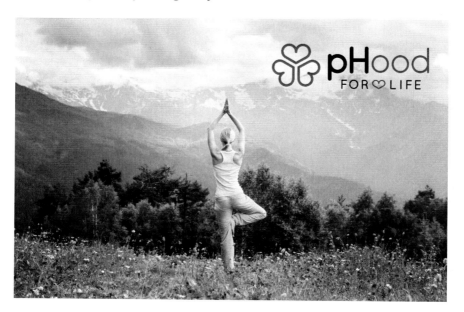

Meditation: Again, apart from aiding in stress reduction, meditation also aids in mindful breathing, which leads to higher oxygen intake and, ultimately, higher pH. Plus, as we talked about earlier, less glucose (sugar) will be released into your system.

Emotional Freedom Technique (EFT): But as finding peace and relaxation while meditating can be easier said than done for a lot of people, it can be even more so when in "panic mode" (such as right after a diagnosis). EFT could be a great alternative or addition. Also known as "tapping," EFT has helped many people find freedom from their stress. It's a form of physiological acupressure in which you tap with your fingertips on certain pressure points to optimize emotional health. Personally, I experienced interesting developments after my journey with cancer and one of them was related to meditation. Before my diagnosis I had an "urge" or "need" to find peace and tried meditation. I found it challenging to relax and not focus on the "chatter" in my head. But after some time into my journey I discovered that I didn't have that "urge" or "need" to meditate much anymore and when I did occasionally sit down for meditation the "struggle" to do it had dissipated. I felt calmer, clearer and more connected in general. I am still not clear on how this change manifested or if it had anything to do with tapping but I strongly recommend this technique for any kind of stress. It is direct and many report instant relief. Check out Bruce Lipton, PhD, or Nick Ortner's *The Tapping Solution* to learn more.

Lists: Another good tip to help reduce stress is to write lists. I often write a list at night of things that I need to accomplish the next day. This de-clutters my mind and helps me sleep better. I also write lists of what I want to accomplish for the year ahead, grouped under different sections such as health, finances, home, etc. Just make sure to not make the lists too ambitious; you don't want to feel frustrated if you don't accomplish everything you've written down.

Yoga: This ancient practice is a wonderful, low-impact way to get the blood flowing in your body. It also rebalances the endocrine system and reduces stress through altering the body's fight-or-flight conditioning. Yoga has often been instrumental in returning cancer patients to their original healthy state, and an Ohio State University study found that women who took just 12 weeks of yoga following breast cancer treatments reduced their fatigue by 75 percent and inflammation by 20 percent. Mainstream medicine still doesn't understand how yoga works so well, aside from increasing oxygen and lowering hormones like cortisol and adrenaline, but yoga also may also reduce the toxic load of the body and send nutrient-rich blood to the places your body needs it most. Yoga boosts the immune system, and for those who understand qi or "chi," also known as prana, this subtle energy is affected profoundly when yoga is practiced, sending healing energy throughout the body, mind, and nervous system.

There are ancient texts that speak of the efficacy of yoga and its sister science, ayurveda, going back tens of thousands of years. When you consider that the type of medicine practiced in the U.S., Europe, and most industrialized nations is only around 400 years old, it makes you think twice about what this system might be overlooking—things that practices like yoga, tai chi, and other systems of movement, combined with breathing and relaxation, might offer. Fellow natural health advocate Christina Sarich, a yogi and writer, told me that yoga has helped her students with ailments as small as the common cold to issues such as diabetes, high blood pressure, and cancer.

Nature: Being outside in nature also heals you. A 20-minute walk in a forest, park, or near an ocean can boost your mood; energize your brain; and reduce hormones that cause anxiety, tension, and sugar cravings.

Walking away: This stress reduction is easier said than done, but it's worth mentioning: leaving situations with people that cause us stress. Toxic relationships can have huge negative effects on health. And it's not just about your partner, relatives, or personal friends. Toxic relationships can also be with colleagues or bosses at work. Again, being willing and able to set boundaries, whether in your personal life or at work, can work wonders for your health.

Summary:

Stress release activities help turn off the stress hormones.

Stress reduction helps to reduce the amount of glucose being released in the body. Glucose is sugar and sugar feeds cancer.

Addressing past traumas is a key ingredient in reducing stress.

10

Detoxification of Your Body and Your Environment

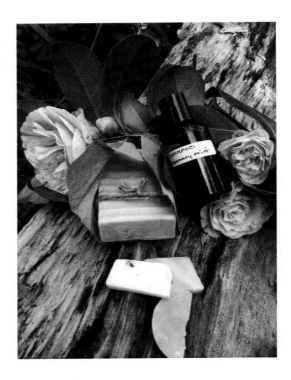

One thing that should not be ignored for better health is the detoxification of the body. This can be accomplished with many different methods or a combination of them. Some of the methods already mentioned in this book, such as the diet, hydration, and juicing, are very helpful for detoxing.

In just two generations, tens of thousands of new chemicals have come into use in industry, in the workplace, and in our homes. At first, the evidence of increases in cancer rates in connection with this increase in toxins was only circumstantial. But now there is well-established science supporting this link. Living without toxic buildup is virtually impossible, which is why our body has a built-in mechanism to deal with a certain amount of toxins. Anything we eat, drink, or even inhale goes through our body's cleaning system. (Lighting a cigarette releases more than 50 known carcinogens into the air—and into the lungs of smokers). Beyond external sources, toxins can also come from normal metabolism and intestinal buildup of unhealthy bacteria within the body itself. Sweating, urination, and bowel movements are all ways in which the body rids itself of toxins. To a certain degree, the body is capable of ridding itself of internal toxins, stress-based toxins, and environmental toxins, but there's only so much it can do. The ever-increasing toxic burden in our air, water, and food from pesticides and chemicals, combined with the increasing stress in our society means our bodies are overwhelmed with toxic buildup and need help expelling unnecessary waste.

Children are often the most at risk as the effects of chemicals are often magnified in children, whose bodies are still developing and changing. The rate of childhood cancers is rising. Cancer is now the second leading cause of death in children, after accidents. A study entitled "Home Pesticide Use and Childhood Cancer" published in the *American Journal of Public Health* showed that there was a direct link between yard treatment with pesticides and an increased risk of cancer in children.

But pesticides and other obvious toxins aren't the only problem. Other chemicals that we come into contact with in frequently may also be harmful. For instance, "parabens" is the general category name given to various preservatives in many cosmetic products and sunscreens. Easily absorbed through the skin, they are endocrine disrupters, and since they can bind to estrogen receptors in women, they could potentially affect estrogen-sensitive functions of the body. Similarly, a substance found in some plastics, bisphenol-A, mimics the female hormone estrogen and has been shown to cause defective cell division during development, even at extremely low doses.

Oxygen is required when the body burns calories to create energy, but that metabolic process leads to the formation of oxygen byproducts known as "free radicals." They cause cell damage that can lead to disease. Antioxidants can neutralize free radicals and prevent much of that cell damage. They may even play a role in preventing cell damage that could be caused by exposure to some environmental carcinogens. Many of the foods described in this book have such antioxidant properties. In 1992, a report by the World Cancer Research Fund and the American Institute for Cancer Research stated, "Evidence of dietary protection against cancer is strongest and most consistent for diets high in vegetables and fruits."

Earlier, we discussed the use of microwave ovens in cooking. Abandoning your microwave may also be good for your detoxing efforts. According to Croft Woodruff, writing in *Microwaves: Modern Miracle or Menace*:

> In 1989, Dr. Hans Ulrich Hertel, a Swiss food scientist, and Professor Bernard Blanc of the Swiss Federal Institute of Technology began conducting extensive research on the effects of microwaved food on humans.
>
> There were non-thermal effects that altered the cell membrane permeability, making cells susceptible to invasion by bacteria, fungi, and viruses. Other adverse effects included the change of cells from healthy aerobic (oxidation) status to an unhealthy anaerobic (fermentation) condition. Anaerobic cells produce damaging free radicals such as hydrogen peroxide and carbon monoxide, which increase the need for neutralizing antioxidants in the body such as vitamins A, C, E, and selenium.
>
> Another problem with microwaving food is the migration of chemicals from packaging into food. To the shame of Switzerland as a democracy, Dr. Hertzel was essentially gagged by Swiss microwave oven manufacturers through the use of trade laws and the courts, and he was threatened with imprisonment. As this was in contravention of the Human Rights Code, Dr. Hertzel was awarded compensation.
>
> According to William Kopp in the *Journal of Natural Science*, researchers experimenting with microwaves at the institute of Radio Technology at Klinsk Byelorussia found that ingestion of microwaved foods caused a higher percentage of cancerous cells in the blood. Such findings caused microwaves to be banned in Russia in 1976: a ban that was lifted after the collapse of the Soviet Union.

Needless to say, I don't use microwaves anymore.

It may be difficult to release years of toxic buildup when you detox for the first time. Unpleasant side effects can include nausea, headaches, diarrhea, constipation, fatigue, trouble sleeping, skin rashes, brain fog, loss of energy, and more, but this will all clear up once you have expelled the toxins. As mentioned earlier, these are all possible side effects of a candida cleanse as well; I experienced several of these side effects myself. Be aware that such unpleasant effects may occur, but remember that they'll fade away and leave you feeling better than ever.

Try not to detox too quickly, as this can place a lot of stress on your body. If your detox symptoms get too severe, try to ease up a little on the methods and take things a bit slower. I learned the effects of detoxing too drastically the hard way. A couple of years into my journey, I discovered that it's a good idea to first cleanse the colon and the kidneys before starting to cleanse the body of toxic buildup. This is because if these organs are clogged, it's harder to expel the toxins from your body. I didn't do a colon or kidney cleanse to start with personally because I didn't know at the time that this would be a good idea; but I'm passing that knowledge on to you so you can avoid my missteps.

Once you become aware of the toxic burden that's part of our modern society, the thought can be a little overwhelming. But it's not all bad news; there are many ways to help the body deal with this less-than-healthy modern environment.

"Curify" Yourself

To help lower your exposure to toxins in your diet:

- Avoid foods high in additives and preservatives.
- Eat organically grown vegetables, fruits, and grains.
- Drink plenty of water in between meals.
- Clean fruits and vegetables using baking soda or apple cider vinegar diluted in some water.
- Cook with cast iron, stainless steel, or ceramic skillets
- Store food in glass containers whenever possible. Alternatively, you can wrap wax paper around your food when storing it in plastic containers to protect against the unhealthy chemicals in plastic.

Jenny Magnusson

To lower the toxins in your environment:

- Wear protective clothing when working with toxic materials.
- Replace furnace and air conditioning filters regularly.
- Choose organic cleaning products and skin products and paraben-free shampoos and conditioners.
- Exchange chemical-ridden air fresheners with incense or natural oils.
- Avoid cell phone radiation by not keeping your phone too close to the body.

Additional Ways to Detox

In the years following my recovery I have learned that there are numerous ways in which you can help your body detox. Now, although several of these are part of my lifestyle today, I haven't tried all of them but still feel that they are worth mentioning as other people have had success with them. They include:

— Adding fiber and fruit pectins to help move toxins through the colon.

— Consuming bentonite clay. Bentonite clay can produce a negative electric charge once it's hydrated, which helps to pull heavy metals, radioactive material, and other toxins out of your body and into your eliminative channels. Should you do one, bentonite clay is helpful to include in a candida cleanse. It's also soothing for the intestines.

— Sweating. Allowing the body to sweat helps the detoxification process. It is therefore wise to not use antiperspirants; instead, choose natural deodorants or nothing at all. You can help rid your body of everything from arsenic to BPA and a host of other unwanted materials by sweating. Get some exercise or enjoy the hot summer sun to trigger this benefit.

— The lymphatic system is our detox machinery. We can help the lymph system through lymph massage, dry brushing, and even rebounding, which allows the lymphocytes to move throughout the body.

— Exercising! Speaking of getting things moving, nothing can be eliminated through the bowels correctly if we don't move. A simple walk while taking deep breaths can help the body to detox.

— Drinking green tea instead of coffee. It reportedly has up to 35 times as many antioxidants as coffee, which also help rid the body of accumulated toxins. (And remember: coffee is acidic.)

— Hundreds of herbs from a diverse heritage of medicinal wisdom and a myriad of cultures efficiently detox the body. Dandelion root, organic gum acacia (from the acacia tree), chlorella, spirulina, milk thistle, black walnut, peppermint, and cilantro for starters. *Cascara sagrada* and wild burdock root are also reported to be effective. Additionally, you can try sarsaparilla. The herb has anti-inflammatory properties to treat the liver, diaphoretic properties, and binds with toxins that are removed from the body through sweating. If you combine any of these herbs with gentle exercise, or a nice hot sauna if you are feeling up for it, you can sweat out lots of toxins.

— Taking hot baths. The skin can release many toxins simply when you're taking a hot bath. Add a little bentonite clay or baking soda and the water will work even harder to detoxify you.

— Drinking more pure water. When you drink pure water, your cells naturally respirate better, meaning less cellular waste within the cells themselves.

— Eating foods high in pantethine, the biologically active form of the B5 vitamin, which can help open blockages created by pesticide consumption. When we are too clogged with pesticides, our bodies cannot naturally detoxify themselves. Broccoli, cauliflower, eggs, and brown rice are all high in pantethine.

— Activated charcoal. Activated charcoal binds to toxins and ushers them to the intestines so that they can be eliminated easily.

— Eating citrus. Skip fruit juices, which often contain too much sugar, and instead add a slice of lemon or lime to your water.

Citrus is a great chelator, helping remove heavy metals and metabolic toxins.

— Eating garlic to boost the production of lymphocytes, a key element to detoxifying through the lymph system.

— Consuming Brazil nuts, which contain glutathione, a natural detoxifying substance.

— Eating dandelion greens. They are known for unclogging the liver and supporting detoxification.

— Put broccoli sprouts in your salad. These little sprouts contain up to 20 times more sulphoraphanes (detoxifying plant compounds) than the full-grown plant.

— Adding turmeric, the Indian spice that comes from a tuberous root. Not only has it been shown to reduce inflammation, but among the many benefits of this spice it is also a great detoxifier.

There! Although detoxing may seem daunting at first, with all of these examples, you are likely to find at least one that works for you.

(And as always, check with your doctor if these are advisable in your specific case).

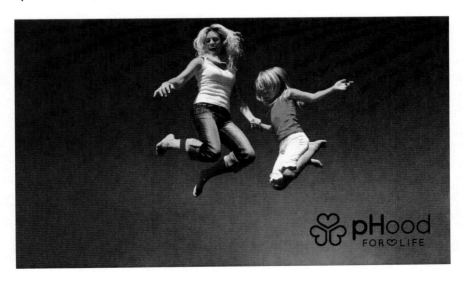

Summary:

Detoxification of the body can be accomplished with many different methods, including juicing, diet, sweating, and hydration.

Antioxidants can neutralize free radicals and help to prevent cell damage.

11

Visualization

Visualization is a powerful technique in any situation. Athletes use it to manifest their preferred outcome, like winning a race or breaking a new world record. This technique is just as powerful for beating an illness. Personally, I visualized that the cancer cells were being gobbled up by my immune system. It may seem silly, but it really helps to put intention into "removing that which makes you ill". You can come up with whatever visual helps you to imagine your cancerous cells being eradicated.

I have for many years worked on improving my Manifestation techniques in all areas of life by working with my five senses, applied for the sake of accomplishing an end goal. The trick is to imagine that you're already there. Imagine the desired outcome as if it is already a reality. Taste it, smell, it, hear it, feel it, and touch it. What does it look like? How do you feel within that reality? Make it real in your mind.

Using this technique, if I wanted to find myself free of cancer or even the fear of cancer, I imagined myself in the surgeon's office and her telling me that there was no more cancer and how it would make me feel when I was told this. I imagined who was there with me. I imagined the smell in the room. Was it was warm or cold? Doing this practice helps to put the focus on a positive outcome in every area of life. The key is to imagine the goal as a reality with *all* your senses. I imagined never being scared of cancer again and how that would feel. Well, I am no longer scared of cancer...and how does it feel? Fantastic!

I guess here is also where the "placebo effect" comes in—in a very positive way. If I believe that something is going to work and help me, it will.

Gratitude and Changing Focus to Change Reality

I am a strong believer that **whatever we focus on grows**. If we focus on the bad things that are going on in our lives, the wrong things will continue to happen, and vice versa. So by focusing on the positive things in our lives, those positive things will grow. My favourite exercise—one that I have used for many years—originates with Anthony Robbins. The version I use amounts to five questions you answer every day:

1. What am I grateful for?
2. What am I proud of?
3. Who loves me and whom do I love?
4. What can I do today to better my life?
5. What is wonderful about today?

Now, in the beginning it may be hard to be grateful if you are suffering, but there is always *something* you can find to be grateful for. Perhaps I am grateful that I can see, or I am grateful for having my legs to walk on, or I am grateful for a happy childhood. The second question doesn't have to be a major achievement; it can be something small like "I am proud of how I handled the situation with that difficult person" or "I am proud that I stayed true to myself and said no when I wouldn't have honored myself by saying yes." The answers to the third question, I've noticed, just keep growing and growing. The fourth question's answer can be something as simple as drinking more water or going to bed earlier. For me, the answer to the fifth question was often that the sun was shining that day. You will be surprised how quickly the list will start getting longer and longer and how your environment and situation start to move in the right direction.

The Power of Prayer

Praying or being prayed for does not require a belief in a particular religion. Energy is everywhere. So is consciousness. Prayer puts clarity and intent into what one wishes to happen. Praying for something works a little bit like stress release when you can leave that stress or worry to someone or something else (the divine, some might say) to help out with.

Vision Board

Those who want to take visualization further can also create a mind map or vision board. I find these very helpful and effective for all aspects of my life. To anyone who thinks vision boards are a joke, consider this: when visualizing, the brain uses the same processes as it does to physically accomplish that task. This means that a bodybuilder can just imagine lifting heavy weights, and the same brain neurons will fire as when he actually lifts those same weights. You can imagine the implications of this, and why visualizing success can be so helpful.

There are several different variations of creating a vision board, but personally, I take a piece of cardboard and then find images, words, and expressions that I cut out from magazines or print from the internet and glue these onto the cardboard. I write with felt pens on the board and add colours that I find appealing for what I want to attract. Once most of the areas on the board I want to improve have been fulfilled, I throw it away and create a new one. So, for instance, if you want to achieve ultimate health, find images that you associate with great health, or perhaps attach your dream body to the board. If you are very stressed, find images that calm you and give you peace, perhaps a plush chair in front of a fireplace, a serene beach with crystal-clear water, or anything that you find blissful. If you are too busy with many responsibilities, find images that you associate with play and laughter. Should you have financial difficulties, you can attach pictures of money and write words such as "wealth" and "abundance" or use pictures of yourself in a time when you *felt* abundant. Your vision board can contain anything that describes the life situation and things you want to achieve that are positive and for everybody's good. You get the idea.

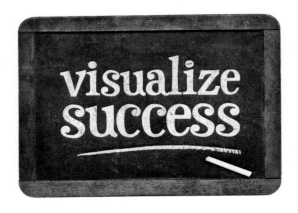

I found some of these techniques helpful in more ways than one: they helped in manifesting a recovery, certainly, but they were also a place to "rest" my worried mind for a while. This is a very welcome thing when you are in the storm of a cancer diagnosis. As mentioned before, many cancer patients have a few months of insomnia following their diagnosis; I was one of those people. I found visualization very helpful on those nights when I woke up in a panic at two in the morning and remembered that I had cancer. I would look at the vision board I created and my mind would find its way back to peace.

Summary:

Visualizing a positive outcome can bring powerful results!

12

Believe in Your Treatment and Be Your Own "Guru"

There's a saying that goes, "I'll believe it when I see it." That never felt right to me. The rearrangement of those words "I'll see it when I believe it" sounds so much better.

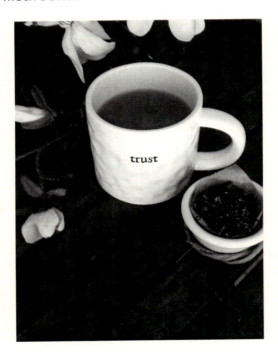

Three months after my diagnosis, and after the pathology report had come back from the surgeon, it was time to talk about hormone treatment with the oncologist. My success with the tumor reduction was ignored; I had refused radiation and now we were arguing about hormone treatment. By now, I was well on my way of understanding how to rid the body of cancer but still didn't know enough about conventional treatments for "prevention." My gut told me that I shouldn't do the hormone therapy, but since I put a lot of faith in one of my natural health connections and, believe it or not, was advised to do it, I agreed to try. I should have followed my gut. I was expected to take the hormones for five years, paying $60 per month. I was told I could expect such things as going into early menopause and aging quicker. After a few weeks on the hormones, I was in such bad shape that I just couldn't take it anymore and once again started researching for answers. I read comment after comment about women having the exact same side effects as me, including cognitive difficulties, memory loss, extreme fatigue, hair loss, and simply not being able to function properly. I knew something was amiss. I then discovered several articles that pointed to that this drug was not proven to be successful at all. In fact, it had been the target of several lawsuits for causing brain tumors, but the companies that created these hormonal "treatments" were only fined a sum of money and then allowed to keep selling them. That's when I stopped taking the hormone pills completely. After this episode, I was more convinced than ever that I know my own body best. I promised myself I would *always* follow my gut from then on and would keep having the courage to take a stand for my own health and for what makes sense, even if it was only to me. I would only follow advice that resonated with me, and would have the courage to do with that information *only* what made sense to me and what felt right. This is when I learned that one should not make gurus out of people, but rather be one's own guru.

Listen. Take inspiration. But always follow your own heart and choose what treatments make sense to you—whatever they may be. This goes for both the natural health field and conventional medicine. When I was first diagnosed, I was very tempted to let an "expert" simply take me by the hand and tell me what to do, trusting in that person one hundred percent, without question. I was feeling vulnerable, emotionally raw, and confused, ready to let someone else deal with the hard choices. I have since come to realize that we are responsible for our own health and our own bodies. We know our own bodies and our own health history better than anyone else. That's why it's important to investigate your own unique case further and do your own research. This knowledge can help you get started, but don't just take my word for it—or anybody else's either. Read, research, ask questions, and take inspiration from as many angles as you can. You may find other variations on the diet that are better suited for your particular type of cancer. Make your recovery your own and take charge of your body. I have found that natural health is also a bit confusing and challenging to navigate sometimes as practitioners

Jenny Magnusson

in the natural health field often don't agree with each other and have different views and convictions. It's extra important in these situations to follow your own gut and the theories you form.

For my part, I didn't know much about cancer—period—when I was pushed and rushed into making a decision about: removing body parts or going through radiation on the day after my diagnosis. The only reference I had to go by were the challenges my mother had struggled with years earlier. I was in a state of shock and I had not had *any* time to do research.

In a situation like that, it's possible to make choices that don't support your overall long-term health. Research and careful consideration can help you gain the knowledge you need to make the choices that are right for you. Take radiation, for instance, which I fought against undergoing. Published in the well-respected *Cancer Journal*, a recent study conducted at the UCLA Jonsson Comprehensive Cancer Center (UJCCC) describes how radiation treatments actually promote malignancy in cancer cells instead of eradicating them. It found that radiation actually encouraged breast cancer cells to form more tumors; moreover, malignancy in radiation-treated breast cancer cells was 30 times more probable than in those not exposed to radiation.

Bear in mind, too that those who undergo radiation are reported to be eight times more likely to develop cancer in their lungs. This happened to my mother.

My doctors didn't tell me any information of this sort. As a matter of fact, I wasn't told much at all about of any of the risks. If I asked about the risks or refused treatment, those risks were downplayed to the extent that it was plain offensive. "Why? Are you planning on becoming an Olympic athlete?" was one of the comments I got from one doctor when we discussed the damage done to lungs by radiation treatment.

Doctors do have an obligation to tell you about the risks if asked, so I advise you to ask away! You can also ask them what they would do in your situation and see if they look you in the eye when they tell you. Does the answer feel honest to you?

It is understandable that we would want to place our wellbeing in someone else's hands. We look to "experts" hoping they will know best, and blindly give our own power away.

94

Doctors are often given a godlike status, which sometimes interferes with respecting our own intuition about what's right for us; it can make us complacent. I feel that we should take our doctors' information and input, but run it through our own intuitive filters and decide whether to apply it or not. The same goes with natural health.

The bottom line is: your body is yours, and your health is yours. They are your responsibility, and you should feel empowered to learn, grow, and take care of yourself in the way that feels right to you.

Summary:

Listen, take inspiration, ask questions, go for second opinions and do your own research so that *you* can make an informed decision for *your* particular situation.

Summary of the Steps

1. **pH Balance**
2. **No Sugar!**
3. **Oxygen.**
4. **Hydration**
5. **Nutrition**
6. **Go Organic**
7. **Gut Health**
8. **Cause?**
9. **Stress Release**
10. **Detox**
11. **Visualization**
12. **Believe in Your Treatment and Be Your Own "Guru"**

Steps that Help Raise pH:

1. Sodium Bicarbonate: Aggressively raises pH, as it has a very high pH in itself.
2. Reducing sugar: Sugar is acidic and avoiding it helps to raise pH.
3. Oxygen: Oxygen, such as through exercise, raises pH.
4. Hydration: Drinking water, particularly water that has a pH greater than the body's pH, helps to raise pH.

5. Nutrition: Eating alkalizing foods help to raise the pH. Certain supplements raise the pH and healthy fats help the body to absorb pH-raising nutrients. Certain oils, like frankincense, help to raise the pH.
6. Gut health: A healthy gut helps the body to stay alkaline.
7. Stress release: A stressed body is more likely to be acidic.

pHood Ideas

What I found most challenging about the Diet to start with was the change in lifestyle it required. For example, I needed to make the majority of my meals myself to make sure I knew what my food contained and how it had been handled and cooked. There are a lot of great recipes out there for alkalinizing food, but since it was already a challenge to find ingredients and the time to cook, I found most of the recipes too complicated, with too many ingredients. My advice is to keep it as simple as you can in the beginning. (I am planning to release a recipe book that you might find helpful, so keep an eye out for it).

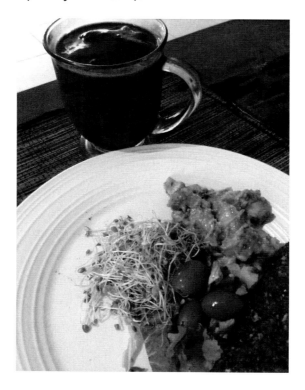

So, to recap a little: raw foods contain the most nutrients, but if your tummy doesn't agree with them now, it might do better a bit further down the road. My stomach is doing much better on more raw food nowadays, but in the beginning of recovery, it's important to consider foods that are easy to digest. Lightly steamed veggies are easier on the stomach. I steamed broccoli or cauliflower frequently in the beginning, and before coming off bread, I would toast sourdough bread, as toasted bread is easier to digest than fresh. Avocadoes seemed to be tolerated easily with a sensitive stomach so I ate lots of those as they also contain plenty of nutrients and healthy oil.

Below are some pHood ideas and some of them might have the words *candida friendly* next to them which will indicate that it's ok to eat after you have gone through the cleanse should you do one. Others might have the words *candida safe* which will mean that you can eat it at any time during your cleanse. Following are just a few ideas that might help you along.

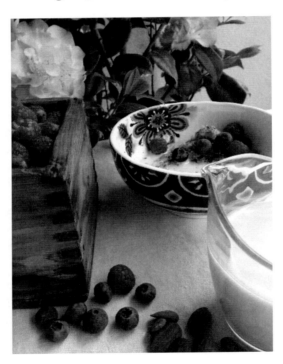

Oatmeal soaked in apple cider vinegar (candida friendly)

Don't fret, it's not as bad as it sounds! This is a breakfast I ate almost every day in the beginning, as apple cider vinegar is alkalizing and good for most anything in the body (with the added benefit of giving you silky-smooth skin). And oatmeal contains fibre and beta-glucans, along with other compounds that help control blood sugar. Oatmeal also contains magnesium. (As mentioned earlier, oatmeal is acidic but the apple cider vinegar is very alkalizing so it helps with that even if the cider is rinsed out.)

Cover the desired amount of oatmeal with water and add anywhere from ½ to 1 tablespoon of apple cider vinegar; let soak overnight. Rinse the oatmeal in fresh water in the morning and add just enough water to cover. Add a bit of stevia and salt. Cook on the stovetop until you have reached the desired thickness. I often add some frozen blueberries. Put in a bowl and serve with almond, coconut, or rice milk. Sometimes I dilute the coconut milk with water if it's too thick. I usually put a little coconut oil, flaxseed oil or butter on my oatmeal to enhance nutrient absorption and sprinkle cinnamon, cardamom, or crushed flax seeds on top. I vary the routine with chopped fruit, dried dates, or sometimes some vanilla drops in the milk. A delicious way to serve your oatmeal involves mixing a few drops of stevia and a squeeze of lemon along with a couple of drops of vanilla into the coconut milk.

Oatmeal is great for regularity as well, as it contains lots of fibre. The "fermentation" of the oatmeal overnight makes it really easy for the body to digest. Should you not be able to stomach the apple cider vinegar part, you can soak your oatmeal in just water overnight, as this still makes the oatmeal easier for the body to digest.

Cottage cheese with flax seed oil (and blueberries)

This is called the **Budwig protocol**. Many people have had success beating their cancer with this protocol alone, as it apparently helps to bring oxygen to the cells. Some people blend the cottage cheese in the blender with a spoonful of flaxseed oil. I prefer to not blend it; instead, I just put some cottage cheese in a bowl with some blueberries (optional) and pour a tablespoon of flaxseed oil over it.

Grapefruit (halved) with coconut milk poured over it (candida-safe)

This might seem like a strange combination, but is delicious—it mellows the tartness of the grapefruit. Grapefruit is chock-full of vitamin C and great for the digestion.

Note of caution: People going through chemotherapy are often cautioned to not eat grapefruit while on the treatment because of its high vitamin C content; this and other cleansing foods are also said to flush the toxic chemotherapy treatments out of the body. Even if you're not on chemo, check with your doctor before eating grapefruit, as before any changes in diet, as it can interfere with certain medications.

Banana mini pancakes

Should you crave pancakes, this is a healthier alternative and a favourite with kids. Best of all, it's very quick! I stayed away from bananas in the beginning of my recovery, as they are mucus-forming, but then slowly reintroduced them. Apart from being alkalizing when ripe, they're a good source of potassium.

1 ripe banana
1 to 2 eggs, beaten
pinch of salt
½ tbsp coconut oil or butter

Mash banana and mix with beaten egg(s) and salt. Pour small amount of batter onto a medium-hot griddle greased with coconut oil or butter. Flip over after a couple of minutes when golden brown.

Topping ideas: mashed figs, raspberries, or blueberries. I often heat up frozen berries in a pot with some stevia and pour over the pancakes. Yummy!

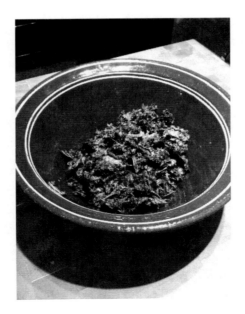

Kale chips (candida-safe)

This is a favourite for most people; even children enjoy these chips. Kale contains much more calcium than milk, making this both a healthy and a tasty snack food.

Rip kale leaves into bite-sized pieces. Massage bits with olive oil and bake on a cookie sheet for 15 minutes or until crisp (but still green) at about 120 C. Season with sea salt.

Sweet potatoes

Sweet potatoes are very alkalizing and can be cooked in the same way as regular potatoes. I often cut them into French fries and bake them in the oven with coconut oil and sea salt. Eat them baked, roasted, mashed, or however you fancy. Another favourite is putting sweet potatoes, onions, carrots, minced garlic, turmeric, celery, and whatever veggies I fancy into a few cups of yeast-free vegetable broth for a quick, filling soup.

Baked root vegetables with onions and garlic

I got hooked on roasted or baked vegetables; they became my comfort food when I needed a change from steamed veggies. You can bake almost any root vegetable and they're great cooked all in the same pan. I almost always roast onions and whole garlic cloves with my vegetables. This technique works well with fennel, beets, cauliflower, carrots, or just about any vegetables that you like (try to stay away from starchy vegetables such as carrots or potatoes if you have candida, though, and then slowly reintroduce them when your body is balanced again).

Cut the vegetables up in chunks and quarter the onion. In a bowl, mix the veggies with a tablespoon of coconut oil (you can melt the coconut oil first if you prefer), a little bit of sea salt, and rosemary or thyme. Bake in the oven until soft but still a bit firm. Ovens vary, but I usually bake vegetables in mine for around 40 minutes at around 170C.

Roasted veggies are yummy with just about any protein of your choice, such as poultry, nuts, or quinoa. I usually put the leftovers on top of a green salad the next day with crumbled goat cheese on top.

Quinoa salad (candida friendly)

This is a great staple salad that is nutritious enough in its basic state, but you can add almost anything to it, such as cooked sweet potatoes, beans, squash, chicken, egg, or nuts and seeds. Use cantaloupe for a fresh summer salad. In the beginning of recovery, you might want to leave out the tomatoes in the recipe. Tomatoes are a bit controversial as they are sometimes referred to as acidic and sometimes as alkaline but I personally stayed away from them in the beginning.

I eat this salad very often when I'm busy, as it also keeps well in the fridge.

1 cup dry quinoa
1–2 cups water or yeast-free vegetable stock
1 bunch of green onions
1 bunch fresh cilantro or parsley
(2 large or 3 medium tomatoes)
juice of one lemon
2 tbsp extra-virgin olive oil, first cold-pressed
Optional: 1 clove of garlic, minced
Optional: fresh mint
Sea salt to taste.

Soak quinoa on the counter in plenty of water for a few hours. Drain, rinse, and cook in 2 cups of water or yeast-free vegetable stock (for flavor) until all liquid is absorbed. Chill.

Finely chop green onions and cilantro (or parsley) and put in a large bowl. Add small cubes of tomatoes. In separate small bowl, combine lemon juice, olive oil, salt, and optional garlic and mint. Pour over tomato mix and toss. Add the quinoa and toss again.

Quinoa contains protein, calcium, iron, magnesium, and vitamins B and E. Cilantro is anti-inflammatory and antibacterial and is effective at relieving nausea and bloating.

Mint promotes good digestion.

Carrot salad

3 large carrots
Pumpkin seeds (I sometimes roast the seeds for extra flavor)

1 tbsp of olive oil (first cold-pressed if available)
juice from half a lemon
1 tbsp of coconut "soy-free" seasoning sauce or tamari

Coarsely grate carrot. Sprinkle pumpkin seeds on top. In a separate bowl, mix lemon juice, coconut seasoning sauce or tamari, and olive oil and pour over. Ready to serve!

Baked peppers with apple cider vinegar and olive oil (candida safe)

Quarter bell peppers. Sprinkle olive oil on top, along with a little bit of apple cider vinegar. Bake in oven for 15 to 20 minutes at 150–170C, depending on your oven. When the peppers are soft but still a bit crunchy and a little bit brown on the edges, they're ready to serve.

Vegetable soup

Since raw foods don't agree with everyone's digestion, including mine, a nice hot vegetable broth does wonders for the stomach (and the soul). You can include any of the vegetables on the list that you like. For those of you who are not vegetarian, using chicken broth or bone broth as a base offers additional healing for the gut (see below).

This is how I usually make my soup:

2 tbsp coconut oil
1 fennel bulb, halved and thinly sliced
1 onion, thinly sliced
2 cloves of garlic
3–4 medium carrots, sliced
½ medium sweet potato or 2 medium beets
½–1 medium zucchini, halved lengthwise and then sliced
4 cups of yeast-free vegetable broth
1 tsp turmeric
black pepper and salt to taste
¼ avocado for each serving
1 slice of lime for each serving
a few twigs of fresh cilantro to top it off just before serving

Cook the vegetables (excluding the avocado and lime) in the coconut oil in large pot on medium/medium-low heat for approximately 5 minutes. Stir often until they start to go a little bit soft. Add the vegetable broth or bone broth and spices and cook for at least 20 minutes or until the vegetables have reached the desired softness.

Serve with avocado slices and a squeeze of lime.

This recipe makes several portions that are handy to freeze.

Whenever I use "heartier" vegetables such as beets, I exchange the lime and avocado with a tbsp of apple cider vinegar and use a diced boiled egg instead of the avocado.

Bone/chicken broths

Bone/chicken broths are very healing for the gut. Bone broth contains amino acids, collagen, gelatin, and trace minerals that help reduce joint pain and inflammation while building strong bones. I occasionally source bones from grass-fed beef and simmer them in water for 48 hours, or chicken feet (organic) for 24 hours. I know it sounds gross, but it really works! I then portion the gelatin-like "jelly" and freeze one portion while using the other portion in the recipe above. If I use beef bones, I add a dash of apple cider vinegar in the soup to give it a malty flavor. If using chicken feet, I add lime juice to take the "edge" off the chicken flavor. I also add some yeast free veggie broth cubes for more flavour to taste. I never have my broths as they are but use them as a base in vegetable soups (see above) as I am not too keen on the taste of only the broth.

Bone and chicken broths have become popular again because of their health benefits and they make the skin softer and nails stronger.

Chicken

If you're not a vegetarian or vegan, there are lots of ways to be creative when cooking with chicken and/or turkey. Although animal protein is acidic and that I am moving more towards a vegan diet, I do still use it—but it's always organic to avoid antibiotics and hormones in the meat. Sometimes I slice the chicken into strips and lightly fry them in a cast-iron pan with coconut oil, turmeric, and salt, then serve with kale that has been tossed in the pan with some coconut oil and minced garlic. These chicken strips are also tasty in wraps with avocado or vegetables.

Another tip is to add some garlic and thinly sliced onion to the pan with the chicken strips, then add some coconut milk and yeast-free vegetable broth powder. Pour over steamed vegetables such as cauliflower, green beans and peppers. Top with chopped cilantro. To make the meal more substantial, I sometimes serve with brown rice or quinoa: yummy and comforting. You can also leave out the chicken if you are vegetarian. I sometimes add some red curry paste and a little bit of stevia. This meal is *candida-safe*.

Flax seed-crusted chicken (candida-safe)

Crushed flax seeds contain lots of healthy omega-3 fatty acids. Store flax seed in the freezer to keep it from spoiling. I put crushed flax seeds on as many things as I can, such as on oatmeal in the morning or on salads, but it's also great for crusted chicken.

Although flax seed has been subject to controversy, some say it affects the production of estrogen and others that it helps the breakdown of it, I have used it a lot with success. Use your own discretion with this.

¼ cup ground flax seed
500g of chicken (breast, thighs, or drumsticks)
coconut oil (for the rack)
1/2 tsp each of dill, oregano, turmeric (optional), and sea salt
1/8 tsp pepper
1 beaten egg

Preheat oven to 200C. Wipe a bit of coconut oil on a rack set on top of a baking sheet.

Mix spices and flax seeds in a bowl. Dip chicken in beaten egg and then in the crushed flax seeds. Place on the prepared rack.

Cook in oven for 20–30 minute or until a thermometer reads 160F (70C) (or until the chicken is no longer pink inside). Serve with a fresh side salad.

Turkey-filled zucchini or eggplants (candida-safe)

2 large zucchini or 2 small eggplants
500–600g organically raised minced chicken or turkey
2 small or 1 large onion, finely chopped
2 cloves of garlic, minced or crushed
extra-virgin olive oil
chopped fresh rosemary, fresh thyme

Cut the zucchinis/eggplants in half lengthwise and scoop out with a spoon, keeping about ½-inch (1+ cm) of flesh on the skin to make the "shells." Keep the flesh and finely chop it. Stir-fry the onion and garlic in a little olive oil in a pan or wok. Add the meat and stir well. Reduce heat.

Add the chopped zucchini/eggplant flesh to the stir-fry. Add salt and herbs; stir to combine.

Once the meat and zucchini/eggplant are thoroughly cooked, stuff the mixture in the shells. Place them in an ovenproof dish and bake for 45 minutes at 175C until golden brown.

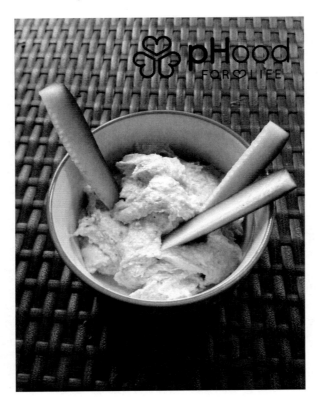

Hummus (candida friendly)

Hummus is an easy-to-make spread/dip that makes a great snack with crunchy vegetables. Chickpeas (also called garbanzo beans) help control blood sugar and contain lots of healthy fiber and protein. Also, should you be loosing too much weight and need some calories, tahini is very high in calories. Below is a standard recipe.

2 cups cooked and drained or canned chickpeas, liquid reserved
1/2 cup tahini (sesame paste)
1/4 cup extra-virgin olive oil
2 cloves garlic
salt and black pepper to taste
2 teaspoons ground cumin
juice of 1 lemon
chopped black olives (optional garnish)
chopped fresh parsley (optional garnish)
olive oil (optional garnish)

Put everything except the parsley and olives, if using, in a food processor and begin to process. Add the chickpea liquid or water as needed to make a smooth puree. Taste and adjust the seasoning. You can garnish with some chopped black olives and olive oil or chopped fresh parsley.

A word on meat

According to Cancer Council NSW, "The World Health Organization has classified processed meats – including ham salami, sausages and hot dogs – as a group 1 carcinogen which means that there is strong evidence that processed meats cause cancer. Red meat such as beef, lamb and pork has been classified as a 'probable' cause of cancer". Processed meat means that it's not sold fresh but has been cured, salted, smoked, or otherwise preserved in some way. Although red meat is rich in protein, iron and B vitamins it is acidic and also contains carnitine. Carnitine hardens the blood vessels and fuels a certain type of bacteria in the gut. Should you be craving meat and absolutely have to have it, try to get wild game meat, as it's free from artificial hormones and antibiotics and it has fed on its natural foods, or bison as it is grass fed. When buying organically raised meat, the cows may still have been fed grains, which are not a natural food for them. Therefore, grass-fed beef, even if it's not organic, may be better for you. It's a challenging maze to navigate, I know, but it deserves to be mentioned. Meat is also hard for the body to digest. I would try to stay away from red meat as much as I could.

How Loved Ones Can Help

Having been on both sides of the fence of a cancer diagnosis, I have gained an understanding of the frustration of wanting to help but not knowing how to approach the situation or what I could actually do to help. Sometimes you can help someone with a cancer diagnosis through something as simple as lending a juicer and buying them some veggies and fruit. Or perhaps you could make a healthy soup that is easy to freeze. Even the most basic chores, such as cleaning, doing laundry, or grocery shopping, can feel overwhelming when you are stressed and sick, so assisting with these things can go a long way to help your loved one.

Listen to and support the decisions of the person dealing with a cancer diagnosis. Yes, you can share your opinion, but don't push for treatment that doesn't resonate with the person suffering. It is stressful enough to be diagnosed; you don't want that person to have to deal with *your* fear, too.

Furthermore, everyone deals with stress differently. Don't take it personally if the person dealing with this diagnosis chooses to talk to someone else other than you. In my case, it was as simple as talking with someone who just happened to be there on a particular day, or during a particular hour, when I was feeling strong enough to talk about it.

Summary:

Lend a juicer

Help source/ buy/ cook healthy foods

Offer anything that makes life less stressful, like helping with chores, babysitting or providing quiet time.

Help source products

Steps Tips

PREVENTION

Nutrition
Hydration
Exercise
Stress Release
(Juicing)
Gut Health

JUST DIAGNOSED

pH Testing
Sodium Bicarbonate if acidic
Nutrition
Hydration
Exercise/Breathing
Stress Release
(Juicing)
Gut Health
Shopping list ideas: pH strips, (juicer, baking soda), greens powder
Remove cause

AFTER SURGERY/TREATMENT/PREVENTION

Nutrition
Hydration
Exercise/Breathing
Stress Release
Juicing
Gut Health
Remove cause

A Typical Day at the Beginning of My Recovery (and sodium bicarbonate for 2-3 weeks only!):

First thing in the morning I had a glass of water

Tested pH on the second urination of the day

Cup of green tea with breakfast (breakfast most often consisted of oatmeal soaked in apple cider vinegar in the beginning of program)

A teaspoon of sodium bicarbonate in a glass of water an hour after breakfast, depending on morning acidity

Glass of greens powder between meals (no set time of day for this)

pH testing just before lunch

Lunch and/or juicing

A second teaspoon of bicarbonate sodium between lunch and dinner if needed

pH testing just before dinner

Dinner

Herbal tea such as chamomile for better sleep

Conclusion

After following my path to recovery, I found myself cancer-free... and candida-free... and all of a sudden, I realized that my allergies were also gone. My eczema was gone. No bloating. I felt healthy and energetic. My weight was naturally balanced and my hair had a healthy sheen and grew more quickly. I had great teeth from having abstained from acidic foods and people started complimenting me on how well I looked. I think it's safe to say that these methods are not just anti-cancerous: they're pro-health.

So, what's the difference between the two bodies, my mother's and mine, that we talked about in the beginning of the book? Well, I think it's obvious to say that in my mother's case, the area around the tumor itself was the focus; and by following the traditional protocol only, she died a painful death in a body that was riddled with cancer throughout despite the treatments. In my case, the whole environment in my body was addressed and changed for the better.

Why We Haven't Heard about These Methods

People are constantly asking me, "How come we don't know about these methods that helped you so much?" I always take a moment to prepare myself because the discussion almost immediately gets political. This is my least favourite information to share of all I've found out. But it is an inevitable topic and needs to be addressed.

Early on in my quest for health, I got the shocking answer to that question: there's too much money involved. Just follow the money. The cancer industry was worth $895 billion in 2008—and that number has not by any means decreased. Greed for money, control, and power has existed all throughout history and still does today. The desire for power and stupefying wealth makes sure Big Pharma is going to use all the tricks in the book to protect their profit. An astonishing sum of $2,500,000,000,000 (that's $2.5 trillion) has reportedly been spent on cancer over the last hundred years, making it one of the biggest moneymakers of all time.

"Big Pharma" consists of some of the largest corporations in the world. Sometimes these companies are slapped with lawsuits for selling a drug that does more harm than good, but the punishment is often merely a fine that amounts to far less money than the profit made by selling the drug in the first place, so there is no real deterrent there. After the lawsuit, they are usually still free to continue selling that same drug! The corporations have the same rights as the individual but not the same responsibilities. Until the corporations are properly made accountable and stopped from behaving irresponsibly, we will never freely and easily have access to the many natural and inexpensive healing modalities for cancer.

No matter what, we always hear that these companies are "searching for a cure" and that their latest drug is going to be the one that eradicates cancer.

As for that "magic pill" cure that they make us believe they are working on and can then sell for unfathomable amounts of money...it is never going to happen, for several reasons. One is that the knowledge amassed over the last century on the *real* workings of cancer reveals that restoring the unbalanced and compromised environment in the body through detoxification with *real* food and nutrition, pure water, and clean air may be the *only* cure—and that's something they will never be able to make into a pill.

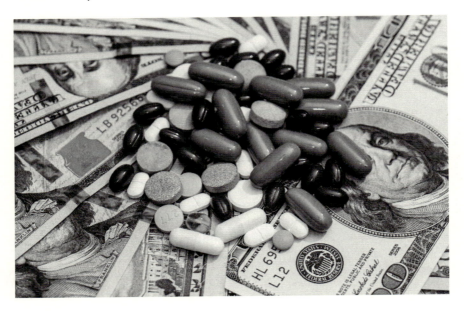

History

How did it all come to this? Well, let's start by going back a century to take a look at some of the explanations that have been presented to me. In the early 1900s, John D. Rockefeller was a giant in the pharmaceutical industry and also owned the Standard Oil Company. (There was and still is a strong connection between synthetic pharmaceuticals and petroleum, as petroleum is often used in the production of pharmaceuticals.) Rockefeller had been convicted of illegal business practices, corruption, and racketeering, but had created a tax haven for himself: the "Rockefeller Foundation," a pharmaceutical investment business. At this time, it was known that vitamins and natural compounds were beneficial to health. But since they could not be patented, Rockefeller's pharmaceutical business could not profit from these beneficial compounds. In a successful attempt to gain control over the medical education system, the Rockefeller Foundation donated large amounts of money to medical schools and hospitals, thereby infiltrating the boards. He also sent a man called Abraham Flexner to the medical schools to write a report, the Flexner Report, which called for standardization of medical education. One effect was that natural treatments with hundreds or even thousands of years of knowledge backing them up were dismissed as quackery. The aftermath of this report resulted in that only allopathy or conventional medicine techniques would be recognized when granting medical school licenses. This resulted in removing education on natural medicine and the biomedical model and thereby also the importance of diet from medical schools. (The control by large corporations also extended to Europe with chemical conglomerate IG Farben, with which Rockefeller also formed an oil/pharmaceutical cartel.)

Hemp, which has been used successfully to treat cancer, was later demonized as it was a threat both as a medicine and as a fuel.

This absence of nutritional education hasn't changed much to this day, leaving us with doctors who are often clueless about nutrition and healthy natural medicine. Today, it is also widely known that doctors for a long time have been courted by pharmaceutical companies to get them to prescribe their drugs rather than suggest healthier options for their patients.

As a result, your doctor might not have an opinion on your diet if you discuss it with him or her, because conventional doctors most often don't have the nutritional knowledge necessary—typically, they've had *at most* 10 days of training on the subject in medical school. I have heard horror stories from doctors who had as little as *two* days of nutritional education offered. And that was optional, and not even required.

I personally don't want to put all my trust into someone making a decision on the nutritional aspects of my health who's had less than a week and a half of training. A common reaction from these doctors who don't have an education in nutrition is to try to deter you from alternative methods altogether. Are they better equipped to give you nutritional advice than nutritionists and natural health practitioners who have studied food and its effects on the human body for years? Should they be able to deter you from trying these natural options without more background knowledge? Don't forget that there are hundreds of thousands of success stories of people having found shining health without stacking up pill bottle after pill bottle, especially when these pharmaceuticals are giving them side effects that even more pills are being prescribed to mitigate. Sometimes people are advised to take these synthetic medications for the rest of their lives. Is that fixing the problem?

To this day, certain trusts are still promoting the pharmaceutical industry, and their influence over medical schools is evidenced in their well-publicized donations to universities. They donate money for *specific* research that ultimately brings them more clout and profit.

To make things worse, Rockefeller included Arthur Hays Sulzberger, publisher of *The New York Times* and one of the directors of the Associated Press, in his Drug Trust. The Trust convinced the Associated Press to not clear any stories on health that had not been cleared by Rockefeller's Drug Trust.

It was suggested in the research I did that this type of criminal suppression of information on real cures around the globe is still a reality today.

In 1913, Rockefeller founded the American Cancer Society. Today The American Cancer Society has net assets of over $1,200,000,000. It is not putting this money into finding a cure but instead works as a tax haven while also helping Big Pharma advance its greed while keeping people in the dark about natural cures. (The American Cancer Society has even gone so far as to try to dissuade from even considering natural treatments such as sodium bicarbonate by previously calling it a placebo on their website. This is just another in their desperate attempts to protect their money-grubbing society.) Let's be clear that their first agenda has never been the welfare of people and a cure for the cash cow. There are a lot of people profiting through this, one of the wealthiest "non-profit" organization in the world, but it just isn't the people one is led to believe profiting from it. It's not the people that are suffering from cancer. For example, in the fiscal year of 2009-2010, their CEO reportedly received over $2 million in salary. My advice would be to put your hard earned money into healthy food for yourself instead of donating to organizations like these.

Clearly, Big Pharma will *never* find a "cure" for cancer. Moreover, cancer is making way too much money for a few multi-national companies for them to let it be known that there are inexpensive, healthy alternatives to their damaging and expensive drugs. Big Pharma is even becoming so desperate that they are printing reports from "respected scientist" that it is dangerous for cancer patients to eat healthfully or to try to balance their body's environment. This would result in people realizing that they can fight this disease and live healthy lives without radiation treatments or chemotherapy drugs. These "respected scientists" are typically working on research projects that are almost always funded by the pharmaceutical companies or private corporations making billions of dollars on their "newly developed" cancer drugs.

After learning all this, I started to understand that the pharmaceutical industry, and the industry to "cure" cancer, are definitely not what they present themselves to be. The champions you are looking for are most often the doctors, scientists or natural health practitioners who have been maligned, defamed, and sometimes even sent packing from their own countries just because they dared to expose the lie or speak up about successful cancer treatments that were not within the "established" medical paradigm.

It is because of the suppression of information that people often don't come across it until they have already gone through treatments such as surgery, radiation, and chemotherapy and been sent home after being told that there is nothing more conventional medicine can do for them. It's not until then, with nothing left to lose, that they find and explore alternative methods. The good news is that many people in this situation have had great success with natural methods, despite starting to use them in the late stages of the illness with more compromised bodies.

In an article in *The New Agora*, physician Dr. Mercola is quoted as saying: "Please understand that cancer is big business. The cancer industry is spending virtually nothing of its multi-billion-dollar resources on effective prevention strategies, such as dietary guidelines, exercise, and obesity education. Instead, it pours its money into *treating cancer*, not preventing or curing it." He also notes that "two out of three cancer patients will be dead within five years after receiving all or part of the standard trinity: surgery, radiotherapy, and chemotherapy. This is not surprising when you consider that two out of three are carcinogenic themselves! One study estimated that chemotherapy benefits about one of every 20 people receiving it."

And further, Dr. Mercola is quoted on the collaboration between the FDA (Federal Drug Administration) and these large corporations, saying: "The FDA is now, thanks to the Prescription Drug User Fee Act (PDUFA), primarily funded by the drug companies and is complicit in this process. They restrict competition in the guise of protecting the public, when the reality is they are protecting the profits of the drug companies."

In addition to this travesty, in 2009, a former VP and head lobbyist of one of the largest Biotech Companies in the World was appointed as deputy commissioner for the FDA—the board tasked with regulating his own industry.

The suppression of information and knowledge about natural medicine hasn't only meant that the public is prevented from accessing this information, but also that knowledge regarding natural medicine that dates back thousands of years in some cases has been almost lost. Another disturbing development is that certain companies that produce natural health products are selling out to big pharmaceutical companies for big bucks, as are certain natural food chains bought up by large "food" companies. In some cases, the smaller natural health companies are then immediately shut down, a threat no more.

The Truth

As mentioned earlier, I am not passing on this information to try to convince those who don't want to know; this would be a waste of their time and mine. I am passing this information on to help those who have doubts about the dangerous methods Big Pharma is subjecting us to and who have a niggling feeling that there might be something to these stories about "miraculous" recoveries.

These "spontaneous remissions" often happen due to the help of people who have been stripped of their medical licenses or sometimes even thrown in jail, though they've saved many lives. The media ridicules them, and calls them money-hungry "quacks ." Who are the real quacks, though? Where is the *real* money going in the "cancer-curing" industry?

Just how much money does this industry—an industry that tells you they are looking for the cure for cancer—really make? Well, estimates show that the average year provides over $150 billion in profit to Big Pharma.

The Pharmaceutical industry often tries to bring focus to a single natural component's potential as a cure in order to more easily dismiss it as not working. That's like removing cancer cells from their environment to test them; it doesn't take into account the complexity of the human organism and experience, so how can it be expected to be a truthful representation?

Let's think through how conventional medicine works.

Approximately 70 percent of conventional medications were copied from nature in order to be able to get a patent on the "medicine." Pharmaceutical companies cannot patent naturally occurring substances (although changes in laws are constantly attempted to make this happen). But if they make a synthetic version of that natural medicine, they can patent it and therefore profit from it. In a lot of cases, this profit is *huge*. The problem is that our bodies are not designed to fully accept or utilize synthetic medications, often leading to side effects. Sometimes these side effects are severe. And sometimes there are several side effects from the same medication. Side effects are very rare in natural medicine, especially when natural substances are taken correctly and in the right therapeutic amount.

Now, the therapeutic amount is another important thing, I found out, when it comes to the battle for natural treatments and medications. The amount "allowed" on the packaging by the various governing agencies, I was told, is often not enough to have a full therapeutic effect—in other words, you're not recommended the correct amount in order for the medicine to have an effect, and so the natural medicine is dismissed as "not working" or even "quackery." As an example, colloidal silver or large doses of vitamin C are very effective as a natural antibiotic in many cases, if the correct amount is taken for the correct period of time and so on. If the knowledge of natural treatments like colloidal silver or a specific dosage of vitamin C had not been suppressed as it has, we could possibly have radically reduced the need for prescription antibiotics and, therefore, potentially reduced or even prevented the emergence of "superbugs" that are resistant to these antibiotics. I have myself had success with both colloidal silver and large doses of vitamin C in situations where antibiotics had been prescribed previously and therefor avoided unnecessary use of them.

This is just one example of many epiphanies I have had along this journey through natural medicine and discoveries that are not just limited to cancer treatments.

The brilliant Dr. Mark Sircus, when talking about natural cancer treatments, states: "It is belittling to medical intelligence to conceptualize one individual medicinal as a cancer cure, since there are literally hundreds of such medicinals, but some are much stronger than others (76)." In Dr. Sircus's book, Dr. Charles Morris is quoted as saying "Eighty percent of your genetic predisposition toward disease can either be activated or held in check by proper diet and lifestyle (75)." Interesting statistics to consider as young people are encouraged to instead remove body parts where cancer *might* show up in their future. The cancer industry exploits our fears.

Charities and Cancer

As if there wasn't enough money made from chemotherapy and radiation treatments along with cancer drugs, the cancer industry makes a killing from hard-working, good-hearted individuals who shell out money in hopes of finding a cure for themselves or the people they love. Even after raising the cost of treatment to more than $100,000 on average—per cancer patient—still *more* money is asked for in the form of donation schemes, often created not by and for morally upstanding organizations. It has been proven again and again that only a small fraction raised actually goes toward any legitimate cancer research; the rest of the money raised typically goes to pay the inflated salaries of staff members, to the next fund drive, or to hospital care. The research that *does* get funded from these donations is not research towards a cure, but research into more sophisticated cancer drugs that Big Pharma can make billions from (or to dismiss the real cures). Knowledge about simple, inexpensive, non-patentable potential cures is simply suppressed.

There are more examples of money raised for finding a cure *not* going towards finding a cure or to help cancer patients. Four cancer charities in the U.S. were recently charged with fraud by the Federal Trade Commission (FTC) for a sham that amounted to over $187 million; among them were the Breast Cancer Society Inc. and the Children's Cancer Fund Inc. The investigation also found that James Reynolds Sr. and the Cancer Fund of America Inc. were using 96 percent in donations they received on themselves or to fund "private fundraisers". They used the funds raised on six figure salaries for family and friends and luxury lifestyles. Funds from these charities were reportedly also used on cars, carnival cruise, meals at Hooters, tax-free college fund, jet-ski rentals, sports tickets and trips to Disney World. These organizations spent at the most 4 cents on the dollar on anything related to cancer.

Inflated salaries in so called "non-profit" is nothing new. The former CEO and president of the Susan G. Komen Foundation for example, made more than $550,000 one year. This cancer foundation also has ties to the pharmaceutical industry.

The links go on and on. National Breast Cancer Awareness Month (NBCAM) was founded in 1985 as a partnership between the American Cancer Society and the pharmaceutical division of a chemical company that is now part of one of the worlds largest pharmaceutical companies. From the start, NBCAM's aim has been to promote mammography as the most effective weapon in the fight against breast cancer. A recently published study in the *Journal of the Royal Society of Medicine* admits that mammography is "a harmful medical practice". The pharmaceutical company in question is the maker of several "anti-cancer" drugs, of which two of them are blockbusters. I was subscribed one of them and this particular drug is actually classified by the International Agency for Research on Cancer as a known human carcinogen.

If you want to learn more about the undeniable ties between cancer charities and pharmaceutical companies, you can check out the works of Samuel Epstein, M.D..

Pharmaceutical companies are simply making billions off pain and good intentions.

In addition to all this, there are many companies that ride the money-grubbing wave by associating themselves with cancer charities. "If you buy our product, we will donate X amount to cancer research," they say. That donation goes to helping prevent you from finding the real truth about how to prevent cancer.

My own experience with donation entities

I e-mailed a woman who was a director at one of those non-profit organizations and asked where exactly the money they raise goes. She immediately took a very defensive stance and proceeded to e-mail me a list of the different hospitals that received some of the donations, never answering my question about what percentage *actually* goes to research or what *kind* of research is being done with the money. After I asked again, giving her an opportunity to address my concerns, she said she didn't want to e-mail the information to me, but rather talk about it over the phone. I called her, but she never took my calls.

I also went to a breast cancer "charity" event and chatted with people about my recovery, sharing what I had found. They were all very interested except one man who got angry with me and said "You are wrong!" and "You are talking to the wrong person!" When I asked why, he explained that he was the husband of the woman who had started the charity. I immediately replied, "Great! That should mean that I am talking to the *right* person, then, don't you think?" Instead of saying "Congratulations! How did you do it? Tell me more. I am sure there are many people here today who want to know more," he angrily walked off.

So is it safe to say that these entities have more to lose than gain if a non-patentable cure for cancer were to be exposed? Many people are still kept in the dark about these things and would rather accuse the natural health advocates of being "quacks" than taking a hard look at Big Pharma. Sure, there are some dubious individuals on the natural health side, too, but that's just the kind of weed one has to navigate through. Keep in mind that the important thing is to stay focused on what makes sense for *you*.

University studies

I wrote the following sentences before the findings of the studies below were revealed: "$2,000,000 was recently given to a lab at a university to study sodium bicarbonate's effect on cancer. The fact that it's been used, tested, and documented to help heal thousands of patients around the world for decades is ignored or suppressed. Why? Well, I'll let people draw their own conclusions and also guess the 'results' the studies at this university will reveal. But to those who discredit many tried and tested natural methods to treat cancer, I can only say: There is no smoke without fire...at least not when there are thousands of us proving that it works. I don't need a university study to prove to me that it works. I know it does. Although I very much doubt that this is what the 'study' will show."

I have since read some of the findings of these studies and surprise! I was right. They found that baking soda's possible effect on certain tissues of the body was "unacceptable!" ...And the effects of chemotherapy or radiation aren't?

I'd rather deal with the consequences of taking a little baking soda than the risks of toxic conventional treatments. For me, any possible risk (and I'm very skeptical there's a real risk at all) to any tissue in my body is *not* unacceptable to me considering the alternative. It would be a small price to pay compared to the damage that radiation, chemotherapy, surgery, and hormones can cause. In any case, we have the right to choose for ourselves what is and isn't acceptable to us. There was also a surprising claim that some cancer cells were found to be alkaline, which is the first time *any* research has noted that, to my knowledge. Again, studies paid for to discredit natural cures. But one only has to put this one question to them: why the interest to do a study on sodium bicarbonates effect on cancer cells at all unless there has been several claims that it works?

Among those whom I have come across who have tried these healing methods, or similar ones, so far, there is not a single person who hasn't reported positive results in one way or another. Pretty good odds, wouldn't you say? To the skeptics out there: Why not try it anyway? What is there to lose? These are natural, harmless methods, if done right.

The conventional medicine "experts" talk themselves into circles and very often contradict themselves. They try desperately to make cancer sound so complicated. In their defense, in some cases, it *is* complex, but for the most part, it is way simpler than they will ever let on. There's a benefit in keeping us in the dark and hiding behind complicated medical verbiage. They'll just assume that we won't question their authority and will continue to spend our last dollar on donations to "find the cure."

As a side note, I think it's also worth mentioning that 70 percent of certain oncologists' income is based on the drugs they are selling.

So, as you might start to suspect, there's a huge monetary benefit to keeping cancer a "mystery" and to suppressing information that lets patients heal themselves.

As a side note to residents of the UK, where I used to live, although "not fully enforced," the Cancer Act of 1939 basically prohibits spreading information on natural treatments for cancer.

"Cancer is just bad luck"

After the discovery of my tumor having shrunk, I was elated and told my oncologist about some of the methods I'd used. He took my hand and forcefully said, "Cancer has nothing to do with diet or lifestyle or any of that. *Cancer is just pure bad luck, Jenny!*"

Cancer rates have increased by 1,500 to 3,000% in under a century—is that how much bad luck has increased too? That is just as absurd as some of the explanations from Big Pharma as to why optimal nutrition and natural health wouldn't be good for the human body, especially in patients who have cancer.

Doesn't it make more sense to take a closer look into what *has* changed in the last century? Such as:

- The rise of fast food
- Less nutrition
- GMO (genetically modified) foods
- Increased sugar consumption
- Pesticides
- The earth being depleted of minerals and nutrients so the crops don't absorb as much
- Less pure water
- Less clean air
- More toxins
- Chemical cleaning products
- Introduction of mammograms that blasts the breast with radiation
- Increased use of antibiotics in humans
- Increased use of antibiotics in animals
- Increased use of growth hormones in animals
- Increased use of steroids in animals
- Increased use of synthetic pharmaceutical drugs
- Birth control pills (hormones)
- More stagnant, sedentary lifestyles
- More time spent indoors (with less fresh oxygen)
- More stressed lifestyles

Isn't it logical to address these areas when talking about the increasing incidence of cancer?

Five-year survival rate

The deeper I got into the research, the more clear it became to me why pharmaceutical companies use the five-year survival rate whenever talking about the "successes" of their drugs. The fact of the matter is that after those five years, the survival rate drops dramatically on conventional treatments, so the companies need yet another complicated explanation to hide behind. To me, it's simple. Unless you don't die from cancer or cancer-related issues such as from treatments *at any time*, you are *not* a cancer survivor. Period. No matter how many years later it is.

Here's some food for thought: With all these billions of dollars in donations over the years, wouldn't you think that they would have made some progress rather than going backwards, with one in every three people (or even worse, 41 percent in some estimates) expecting to get cancer today, rather than estimates of one in every 40 less than 100 years ago? (And these are figures the companies use themselves whenever it suits their needs to scare people into parting with their money).

Cancer and the Media

To make matters worse, you aren't able to just do an easy internet search anymore and find information like this unless you really dig for it and know what you are looking for. The large corporations and donation entities that don't want you to hear about it have the money for this kind of information being controlled in various ways and not being spread to the masses. Their money will for example ensure that their sites, information and disinformation show up at the top of searches.

When I started my research on these methods a few years ago, it was fairly easy to find the information I was looking for. Sadly, it is getting harder and harder nowadays as a lot of information has also been removed. An example of this kind of activity is that an entire top natural health site of a reported 440 000 pages was removed by Google without warning. Poof! Apparently it was on a minor technicality that definitely shouldn't have brought down the whole site (and that other large mainstream news sites were also doing but were left alone). Other reports stated that there was no rational explanation whatsoever from Google of why they took the whole site down. Whatever the reasoning for this action was, Google is a private company after all and money talks. On a positive note, because of the large vocal backlash against Google's delisting, the site was restored a few days later and had also sparked new discussions and debates about search engines, censorship and free speech according to the owner of the site.

Advertisements for drugs make up for a large number of the TV ads. This is one of the reasons why TV stations typically don't air honest information and programs about alternative cancer treatments, as they are in essence controlled by these companies' money. This is why unless you hear it directly from a friend or pick up a book like this one, you probably won't learn that an alternative treatment for cancer exists. Big Pharma's websites get top billing on search engines because *theirs* tell the story they want told—and they say it's based on facts. Who decides what is fact and what is fiction when the other side—namely those treatments that cannot be patented for big bucks—have not been properly funded, supported, or tested? Stopping information is only logical when it is a threat, because if it were nonsense, they wouldn't have anything to lose by allowing it to be spread. The reasoning for stopping the information to be spread is often "to protect people from being harmed by natural methods". Hundreds of thousands of people die every year from conventional "treatments". And what about the freedom of speech, freedom to choose what to believe and freedom of choosing what I decide for my body?

In my case, it took lots of time and effort to find out the real truth about getting free from cancer when I could have simply been given these choices and focused on getting better.

If we all lived in the era when scientists were saying that the earth was flat, you can imagine what would have showed up in the top spot on Google when searching for information on geography.

The large corporations also have the money to employ people whose sole task is to discredit information on the internet. You may know it as "internet trolling." After I had learnt more about the truth and the people who wrote about it I started to notice a common theme from the corporations "trolling". There would be comments posted regarding the links to the very helpful books and articles I had read with phrases like "He claims..." or "he is not a doctor..." or "there is no scientific evidence to these claims" or even worse the constant use of the word "quack" but it was obvious that most often the poster hadn't even read the piece. This is of course a very effective way of keeping people from even bother opening the link. The short of it is that Big Pharma is trying to convince you that the earth is still flat. They use scientific "evidence" to support their opinion while telling you that there is no scientific evidence that the earth is round, just as in the time of Copernicus, all to keep you from seeing the true, big, wide (round) world of possibility.

Real Quacks and "Orthorexia Nervosa"

The true cure for cancer is not something that can be patented, and if it can't be patented, it will be tested improperly in order to make it fail and discredited. This is all done in the pursuit of money and power. It sounds sinister—and it is.

Good nutrition and good health pursued through a natural approach (and one compound in particular) are a threat to Big Pharma for obvious reasons. Furthermore, the pharmaceutical companies are very scared of having the enormous lies they've been telling exposed, and are using more desperate ways of keeping their very profitable untruths hidden. One of those ways involves claiming that those of us who have discovered other ways of beating illness, which also happen to be better for the planet and its other inhabitants, are "crazy" people who suffer from a mental condition they have named "orthorexia nervosa." It really is laughable.

Another way to protect themselves is by twisting the actions of natural health into "quackery," and saying that anyone selling "natural cures" is "money grabbing." This is projection. The money being made in natural health in comparison to Big Pharma is miniscule. Big Pharma is the *real* quack. Most natural health advocates risk their money, work, and reputation by telling the truth, since they can't hide behind anonymity as Big Pharma does. This anonymity is also often evident in the websites you will find on the highest spot on Google above the websites that are exposing the truth. The ones exposing the truth are typically real people with their names included. The ones trying to stop you from reading it are usually hiding behind anonymity, originating from companies that have a lot to loose if you happen to read and believe in these truths. If anyone thinks fame and fortune drive people to tell the truth about natural health, they should think again. I'm mentioning this to again to be mindful of where the information is originating from and what resonates with you. A tip is to scroll down a little bit on your search pages and read the conflicting information and then listen to your gut and what's resonating with you. If the conventional explanation still "wins" then so be it, but then you have at least put your "gut" to the test.

Sure, there are people who don't make it on natural medicine regimes as well, naturally (then again, I don't know of anyone personally). On conventional therapies, however, I know of plenty of people who didn't make it, and that's after suffering terribly. And the ones who did make it on conventional treatments experienced some kind of side effect, if not considerable suffering.

In order to be entitled to dismiss people as quacks, shouldn't you be required to experience the situation yourself? In my view, you should have had cancer yourself first and tried these methods personally. If not, you might be preventing people from getting access to lifesaving information. If they don't want to hear it, there are those who do.

Offensive remarks such as "conspiracy theorist"

I can honestly say that I am sick and tired of defending these methods when faced with skepticism. But more than this, *I am sick and tired of cancer.*

A good quote on this subject comes from Dr. Mercola: "We've all heard the label 'conspiracy theorist,' which is the most popular label used when an idea or story is unfavorable to the mainstream media and the interests that back them up. You are a 'conspiracy theorist' if you ask questions, assimilate facts in a logical manner, or pursue justice outside of the main flow of public discourse on a popular issue."

Dismissing those of us that have discovered the truths about the cancer industry and natural health as a "conspiracy theorist," is very offensive but a very common insult.

I saw my loved one die in a body butchered by conventional medicine and I was personally faced with the possibility of the same destiny. I didn't just get by without Big Pharma's control, but entered a new life of freedom and gained an understanding of my body and how to attain better health with my organs still intact. So, if anything, you can call me a conspiracy *realist* when it comes to the big cancer cover up.

You are the one in charge of your body despite of the corporate cover up. *You* are also the one responsible for your own health, as no doctor or pharmaceutical company will be held responsible for any side effects or damage done to your body by chemo, radiation, surgery, or hormones, even if it kills you (as long as they are following protocol). Natural health practitioners on the other hand, are frequently held responsible for any treatments that are not successful. How is that fair?

Once you have reclaimed your health, be prepared to encounter some dismissive glances or blank stares. Be prepared to be expected to defend yourself when that's not your responsibility. Be prepared to even encounter some angry people who tell you you're wrong even though you have been to hell and back and are standing in front of them, not only still alive but with glowing health. Be prepared to be told you are gullible, when gullible is the very last thing one is when you refuse to keep getting fooled by the Big Pharma paradigm anymore. It was even hinted a couple of times that I was "seduced" into these methods. Rest assured that there is nothing seductive in having to go it alone and try to keep the faith despite being faced with so much skepticism (while at the beginning also having to deal with your own disbelief and skepticism and facing some hard choices). One is so very alone in the beginning of choosing the natural route. That is not seductive. The seduction lies with the traditional side of health, where it is "easier" to just put your life in someone else's hands and let them lead you away and make your choices for you, especially when you are at your most vulnerable, such as after a cancer diagnosis. It is also *very* seductive to find support in the many charities where cancer patients find comfort in each other. It is at that moment when the pharmaceutical companies come in to cash in on ones' vulnerability and empathy.

Be prepared to also hear that "it's not right to give false hope to people." Yes, I have also been told this. How on earth can anything be more *real* hope than this? Besides, I think I speak for most people who have had cancer when I say: when you have cancer, there is no such thing as *false* hope. There is just hope. Plain and simple.

As far as I'm concerned, the false hope is in the conventional "treatments" or in making us think that our hard-earned dollars will go toward *real* research into finding a cure.

Let me just make an important point, though: so far none of these offensive remarks have ever come from a person who has, or has had cancer themselves. And the very worst of the remarks have been from people whose salaries in some way are linked to the cancer industry.

But it's worth it!

Just know that the liberation one feels after having left the old way of conventional sick-care and entered the new of *real* health and awareness is worth every (skeptic-fighting) minute! Moreover, along the way you will start to find your *own* peers. The ones who have found a way out of being a victim of Big Pharma. You may find that there are hundreds of thousands of us, even millions who have found the truth of what *real* health really means. By this, I don't just mean physical health, but also seeing the world through healthy eyes. The focus should be on the health of the planet, on *real* healthy food, healthy water, healthy air, and healthy thinking, and not on profit.

With all this, I'm not saying that conventional medicine doesn't have its place. It absolutely does (particularly in emergency medicine). It's the part of Big Pharma's focus on *profit*, especially in the cancer industry, the *suppression* of information and the *disempowerment* of the patient I'm talking about.

Good doctors

Having said all this, I also still believe that the majority of health care providers and doctors are good people who are doing everything they know how to in order to help their patients get well. My own family doctor was astonished about my progress and asked me about the methods I used so that she could forward some ideas to other patients of hers. This is how your doctor *should* react to your progress: with interest and support. If your doctor is not interested in or supportive of your desire to take charge of your health, change doctors or, at the very least, go for second opinions and research your options.

This is also good practice when dealing with the natural health side of things. I learned the hard way to trust my intuition when a holistic coach suggested that I go ahead with the hormones that my oncologist had advised me to take for the next five years. The coach said it could give me "an edge." I wasn't entirely comfortable taking them once I started to unravel some disturbing information about conventional treatments and learned about the negative effects of the hormones from other patients. But since I'd had such great success with other information this otherwise amazingly gifted coach had given me, I trusted her blindly and started taking them. The effect they had on my wellbeing was devastating and after a few weeks of being incredibly tired, losing cognitive skills, and starting to lose my hair, I dug deeper in my research and found some shocking information about this particular drug and immediately stopped taking it. I have since learned to always do what resonates with me and not blindly follow someone else's advice just because I respect their opinion.

I'm not saying that your doctor is in on the Big Pharma scheme. On the contrary: I am positive that most medical practitioners enter the profession with an urge to help people and save lives. At the same time, one has to take a hard look at how little emphasis is placed on nutrition and its effect on the body in medical schools, and also what drives a practitioner to make certain decisions. Keep in mind that doctors have frequently been bribed by pharmaceutical companies with, for example, exclusive all-expenses-paid trips to the Caribbean and other untoward ways of promoting their drugs and "therapies." Although, there have been some regulatory changes to prevent paid trips and exorbitant gifts to doctors in the past decade.

Furthermore, medical insurance is very expensive for most people in the US for example, and many have no insurance at all. Big Pharma is also in league with these insurance companies. That is why insurance doesn't cover nutritional counseling or other non-traditional methods, even though they work—this would be an admission by the medical establishment (which includes huge insurance companies) that cancer can be cured naturally and inexpensively. And since nearly all hospital revenues come from patient insurance, hospitals will not take the chance of using a substance that hasn't been expressly put forward by the medical establishment.

With the methods in this book, you are your own health insurance, and in many cases, treating your cancer will become much more affordable. For instance, although organic, non-GMO foods cost more, baking soda costs just a couple of bucks. Walking and breathing doesn't cost money. Learning about these methods won't cost you much either, (apart from some anger and frustration over the pharmaceutical companies' gall).

There *are* many wonderful doctors out there who have started to understand the importance of nutrition and who have the courage to support their patients in taking charge of their own recovery. These doctors are partners in helping their patients to make their own choices, even when their hands are tied, as, by law, they are not allowed to stray from the conventional methods taught in medical school. The threat of being stripped of their licenses and/or sued for malpractice is too great. I feel for these people, as it must be frustrating to see their patients suffer. However, I also feel that they have a responsibility to support and speak up for patients in whom they have seen great progress. It is their duty as someone who purports to be interested in healing to spread this information to others that it may help. This should not be too much to ask, as they have taken an oath to "do no harm."

Staying the Course

Learning all this information can be overwhelming.

I have come to realize that the trick for me was (and still is) to wake up and stop being naïve without getting cynical or overwhelmed. I needed to find my peers and get educated on the goings-on within corporations while still keeping my focus on true health and good intentions. And I have thankfully found many people who have had the same experiences I did for validation and support.

I believe that one of the reasons behind my health successes is that I didn't resist the shift. I stayed open.

After following these steps and changing my lifestyle and way of thinking, can I be sure that my cancer will never return? Of course there are no guarantees. I am still struggling with cancer-causing issues, such as not being able to exercise properly due to injury, water issues, missing lymph nodes, unforeseen personal stress factors, and the fact that that I had my chest blasted with radiation several times every six months for mammogram pictures before I was diagnosed and knew better, among many other factors. But to put things into perspective: that is life, and the same would have been true had I gone with conventional treatments. The difference is that after walking my path, my organs are undamaged and my body parts (except for three lymph nodes) are still in place. I haven't gone into early menopause or put even more toxic stress on my body. I have enjoyed good health and energy during the five years I was supposed to have been taking those hormones. In short, I have had a far better quality of life than my mother did at this stage. And to put things into perspective: every person I have spoken to who was diagnosed after me and who went through with the conventional treatments that I didn't use, has said that they regretted it—and some have already been diagnosed with cancer again in a different part of the body.

Start simply

My advice would be to not take on too much, too soon. Although the steps I outline in this book make up a path toward health, you might not necessarily want to try to change everything all at once. Instead, be aware of how many ways you can help your body heal and/or protect itself against disease. Start simply and with the most pressing areas: quit sugar and hydrate properly with a couple of liters of pure water daily (between meals). If you have cancer and a very low pH, I would personally try the baking soda method immediately for a couple of weeks and work myself through the list as I move forward. Whatever works for you.

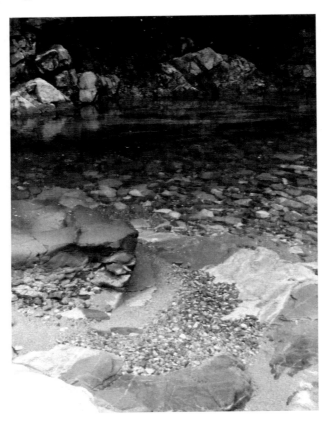

Feeling better and focusing on real health for oneself and the planet

After my journey with cancer and learning about Big Pharma medicine vs. natural health and its practitioners, I have often reflected on it all. I feel it's important to point out that not only was the proof in the pudding when my tumor shrank and the pieces of the puzzle fit the explanations as to why, but it also resonated on a deeper level with how much better I was feeling every day and the gut instinct that *this* was *real* medicine and these people (natural health practitioners) really *wanted* me to get better. They felt so passionately about this that many of them gave me their time free of charge on an already low income while constantly facing ridicule or even banning from their profession.

I find the truth about how to kill and prevent cancer quite amazing, and if you are a person of faith, isn't it interesting that one of the most powerful treatments for cancer is not only natures own but actually one of the most inexpensive and harmless substances around? It's within reach for the poor. And the foods and the products that promote real health are also healthier for the Earth. Now that is a true miracle.

Now that you've reached the end of the story of *my* journey, I hope you will endeavor to start your own. As you will likely find out, healing yourself from cancer also leads to having a healthier mind and body overall. I found this out through my own research and experiences, but I urge you to do your own research, outside of just reading this book.

Ultimately, I don't want you to take my word for it. I just want to be a tour guide who shows you some secret paths to better health that you can meander along on your own time. Do your own research, but be mindful of where any conflicting information comes from. It's important to keep an open mind and think logically through what's behind any given treatment and why it's being promoted.

I went the holistic route, against the prescription of traditional medicine, but I also had a couple of hiccups caused by blindly trusting certain professionals even in the natural field; this led me to make a few choices that I wouldn't have made after conducting my own research. Always remember that you have choices. The medical establishment will pressure you into making quick choices, but take a moment to feel in your gut what seems right for you and what makes sense. Try to remember that most people were feeling just fine when they were diagnosed with cancer, but a few months into conventional "treatment," most people feel and look really *sick*! Does that make sense to you? It doesn't to me.

Don't panic if your doctors give you a surgery date that feels too late for you. There's a positive side to this: you will have more time to get on top of your alkalizing methods, work on de-stressing, and start detoxifying your body. And it will give you more time to make an informed decision. And that informed decision may still be to go ahead with surgery (for example, you may find it may be advantageous, even if you are using alternative methods, to remove tumor burden and make a bit easier for the body to deal with the rest, as this has been suggested in some of the information I have come across from natural practitioners as well).

Remember that your health and recovery are *yours* regardless of what you choose as your treatment, and even if those decisions are not supported by the mainstream medical establishment, your friends, or even close family members. *You and only you know what is best for you.* As you recall, not even my doctor was familiar with the methods I used to shrink my tumor, so you can also imagine that people who have never faced a cancer diagnosis might not be the most informed about the subject either, even if they want the best for you.

Ultimately, you will have to weigh all the theories on your own and make your own health choices. Don't let anyone else make them for you. Empower yourself and be your own "guru." Take inspiration from other people, doctors, patients, naturopaths, and whatnot, but always make the decision *yours.* Remember that your body *wants* to heal.

A cancer diagnosis may not seem like a gift right now, but it is. It is a wake-up call to love yourself more, to learn about how to achieve greater overall health, and to look some of your worst fears in the face and overcome them. No matter what challenges we face in life, it helps to know that others have faced something similar and come out victorious on the other side. I'm not the only person who has beaten cancer at least once in a very healthy way, but you can now add me to the list of people you know who can really sympathize with what you are going through and who also see that you have the strength to overcome the challenges put before you. You can do it!

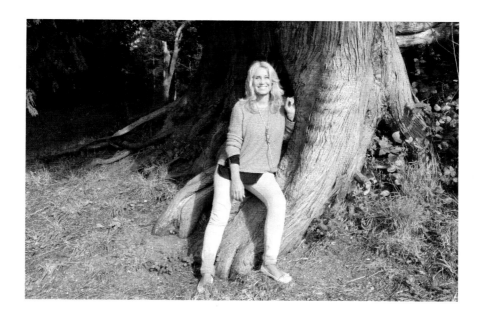

Be well and remember I am here every step of the way in support of your healing, whatever you choose to do.

And whether you are facing a health challenge or not and are reading this book: Let us join together for a better future of our health and that of the planet.

> **"The people that say it can't be done shouldn't interrupt the people doing it."**
>
> — *Chinese proverb*

Resources

To learn more visit: www.phoodforlife.com

Ty Bollinger

After I had nearly finished this book and started to film interviews with subjects from my book and journey, I came across a video series called *The Truth about Cancer* by Ty Bollinger. I was blown away by the research and all of the experts and "cancer conquerors" that he had included in this incredibly extensive series. I have only given you snippets of the going-ons behind the cancer industry's criminal activity and how natural treatments work from my own angle. Should you want to find out more about Big Pharma and where their massive profits originate, be sure to check out Bollinger's information. He's a brave warrior against the corporate domination and the lies about cancer that we are being subjected to.

Strongly Recommended Reading:

- **Dr. Mark Sircus:** *Sodium Bicarbonate: Nature's Own First Aid Remedy*
- Investigative journalist and Pulitzer Prize nominee **Jon Rappoport** has extensive information to share regarding the cancer cover-ups and the frauds perpetrated by the large pharmaceutical companies.
- **Dr. Mercola**
- **Joe Dispenza**
- **Bruce Lipton, PhD**
- **Nick Ortner "The Tapping Solution"**
- **Patrick Quillin, PhD**